SAVING WILDLIFE

The Extraordinary Life and Legacy of Dr. Kurt Benirschke

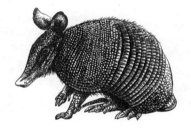

Rolf Benirschke
with James Lund

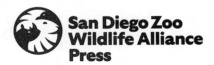

Saving Wildlife: The Extraordinary Life and Legacy of Dr. Kurt Benirschke was published by San Diego Zoo Wildlife Alliance Press in association with Beckon Books. Through these publishing efforts, we seek to inspire readers to care about wildlife, the natural world, and conservation.

San Diego Zoo Wildlife Alliance is a nonprofit international conservation leader committed to inspiring a passion for nature and working toward a world where all life thrives. Its work extends from San Diego to eco-regional conservation "hubs" across the globe. San Diego Zoo Wildlife Alliance supports cutting-edge conservation and brings the stories of its work back to the San Diego Zoo and San Diego Zoo Safari Park—giving millions of guests, in person and virtually, the opportunity to experience conservation in action.

San Diego Zoo Wildlife Alliance Mission: To save species worldwide by uniting our expertise in animal care and conservation science with our dedication to inspiring passion for nature.

San Diego Zoo Wildlife Alliance Vision: A world where all life thrives.

Paul A. Baribault, President and Chief Executive Officer
Shawn Dixon, Chief Operating Officer
David Miller, Chief Marketing Officer
Lianne Hedditch, Vice President of Communications
Georgeanne Irvine, Director of Publishing

San Diego Zoo Wildlife Alliance
PO Box 120551
San Diego, CA 92112-0551
sdzwa.org | 619-231-1515

San Diego Zoo Wildlife Alliance's publishing partner is Beckon Books, an imprint of Southwestern Publishing House, Inc., 2451 Atrium Way, Nashville, TN 37214. Southwestern Publishing House, Inc., is a wholly owned subsidiary of Southwestern Family of Companies, Inc., Nashville, Tennessee.

Christopher G. Capen, President, Southwestern Publishing House
Kristin Stephany, Director of Partner Development
Kristin Connelly, Managing Editor
Betsy Holt, Publisher
Vicky Shea, Senior Art Director
Scott Ramsey, Cover Designer
Jill Scehovic, Proofreader
swpublishinghouse.com | 800-358-0560

Copyright © 2022 San Diego Zoo Wildlife Alliance

Quoted conversations have been faithfully rendered as the author and others interviewed for this book remember them.

All photos © San Diego Zoo Wildlife Alliance, except the following images, which are © Benirschke family: p. 151, 152a, 152b, 153a, 153b, 154a, 154b, 154c, 155a, 155b, 157a, 161b, 163b, 165b, 166b; p. 259b: © Jerry Coli | Dreamstime.com

Back flap jacket photo: © Rolf Benirschke

Illustrations by Anastasia Osipova: AnastasiaOsipova/Shutterstock.com

All rights reserved. No part of this book may be reproduced or transmitted in any form or by any means, electronic or mechanical, including photocopying or recording, or by any information retrieval system, without the written permission of the copyright holder.

ISBN: 978-1-935442-81-3 (hardcover)
ISBN: 978-1-935442-82-0 (softcover)

Library of Congress Control Number: 2022935805

Printed in Canada
10 9 8 7 6 5 4 3 2 1

For my mom, whose quiet strength and endless encouragement supported my dad and inspired us all.

FOREWORD

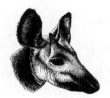

Two Steps Ahead

When I met physician and renowned San Diego Zoo conservation scientist Dr. Kurt Benirschke in 1974, I was a graduate student, still trying to determine my scientific path. I soon realized what so many came to know: that this man of astonishing curiosity, energy, and intellect was devoted to uncovering the mysteries of medicine, genetics, wildlife biology, and much more—and that he would generously give his time and knowledge to anyone willing to learn.

Kurt Benirschke had a warm, engaging personality and treated everyone with compassion and respect. He was a man who cared deeply about solving medical challenges for both humans and wildlife, and he cared just as deeply about his colleagues, friends, and family. He became a mentor and even a father figure to me, pointing the way to my future career and encouraging me every step of the way. It has been one of my goals in life to emulate his commitment, generosity, and thirst for knowledge.

Dr. Benirschke's passion and extraordinary vision shaped developments in reproductive medicine and conservation biology in the latter part of the 20th century, and the impact of his work continues today. The discoveries he and his colleagues made during his tenure at the San Diego Zoo advanced knowledge in wildlife health, breeding biology, genetics, and more, leading to conservation successes for Przewalski's horses, California condors, giant pandas, and rhinoceroses, among many others. His interests, which spanned diverse fields, were unified in his advocacy of One Medicine—the precursor to the integrative concept of One Health, which is now gaining prominence. Many students and scientists he taught and influenced now address urgent issues of our times, such as the global coronavirus pandemic and the conservation of biological diversity.

Kurt was an ardent believer in sharing knowledge, and I remember him telling me, "In the end, all you have is what you have published." His legacy lives on through his vast number of works. Testimony to his influence and impact can be seen in the scientific journal articles, books, and chapters of books he wrote, from his text on the placenta that is still used in medical schools today to published scientific discoveries in biology and genetics that continue to inform the conservation of endangered species.

Yet none of these tributes addresses the full measure of the man. It takes the insightful view of his offspring—in this case, his youngest son, Rolf—to bring the totality of this unique individual to light. Interwoven in these pages are personal reflections that reveal an amazing life and the earned mutual respect, appreciation, and genuine love forged between a father and son.

For me, reading this book brought back rich memories of the infectious enthusiasm that permeated the many wonderful discussions Dr. Benirschke and I had during the decades we worked together. We delighted in speaking of "ideas" and where they might lead us. A good idea shared between us was the oxygen for our work. If that disrupted the status quo and called for engaging new perspectives, we weren't concerned. We knew the world was changing and that scientifically based reasoning was the path that would lead the San Diego Zoo—now San Diego Zoo Wildlife Alliance—to a position of conservation leadership.

The building where the San Diego Zoo first made space for Dr. Benirschke's research department has been refitted multiple times. But the long staircase inside with its low steps that we traversed many times a day remains, reminding me that Dr. Benirschke always took those stairs two at a time. That was how he lived his life—two steps at a time. He was almost always two steps ahead of everyone else, whether in the lab exploring a medical problem or in his Zoo office weighing a decision that would impact wildlife for years to come.

I'm grateful I had the opportunity to witness the enthusiasm, passion, and dedication of this extraordinary physician-scientist and to work alongside him for four decades. His remarkable life is still influencing our world for the better. Enjoy this inspiring read.

Dr. Oliver Ryder
Director of Conservation Genetics
San Diego Zoo Wildlife Alliance

A Note from Rolf

My dad saw a great deal of change during his lifetime—through World War II and in medicine, research, and wildlife conservation. He was a curious trailblazer, always asking questions, seeking answers and new approaches, and pushing the limits of what was possible. His history is best viewed in light of the times he lived in and the knowledge that was available at the time. Standards, practices, and approaches around wildlife, collecting tissue samples, and more—methods that were accepted and commonplace in the 1950s, '60s, and '70s, and even up to a decade ago—have evolved considerably. Some of the stories in this book about Dad's work and my own childhood might seem unconventional because we now do things much differently. Back then, Dad used his ingenuity as well as whatever resources were available to learn and to advance science. I hope, as you read this book, you will view the stories we tell through that lens. That's the nature of change: as we learn more, we apply our new understanding and we take the next steps. Dad knew that, and he was often first in line and always willing to learn, adapt, and move forward. Today's standards, regulations, laws, and attitudes are the result of decades of progress. We now, thankfully, see animals and wildlife conservation in a different light, with an urgency that Dad recognized way back then. I have no doubt that if Dad were still alive, he would be leading us all as he applied this new knowledge and way of communicating and collaborating. He would wholeheartedly approve.

Contents

Prologue: 1969, Tierpark Berlin 1

Part 1   **Germany: Signs and Inclinations**
    Chapter 1: Storm Clouds over Glückstadt 9
    Chapter 2: Death and Life 15
    Chapter 3: Carpe Diem 25

Part 2   **Boston: A Growing Brood**
    Chapter 4: Making a Start 35
    Chapter 5: Grand Rounds . . . and Rings 43
    Chapter 6: Little Zoo on Bird Hill 51

Part 3   **Hanover: Animal Tales**
    Chapter 7: The Kingdom 63
    Chapter 8: Counting Chromosomes 71
    Chapter 9: A Grand Expedition 79
    Chapter 10: Moths and Armadillos 87
    Chapter 11: Ahead of His Time 93

Part 4   **San Diego: One Medicine**
    Chapter 12: California or Bust 101
    Chapter 13: Connections 109
    Chapter 14: A Vision and a Leader 123
    Chapter 15: Give Me a Problem 133
    Chapter 16: A Frozen Zoo 143
    Chapter 17: One Medicine 167

Part 5   **Worldwide: Advancing Knowledge**

Chapter 18: A Pain in the Gut 181

Chapter 19: Proyecto Taguá 195

Chapter 20: Saving Wildlife 207

Chapter 21: President Benirschke 215

Chapter 22: New Hope 223

Chapter 23: A Unique Individual 233

Epilogue: Legacy 247

Afterword by CEO Paul A. Baribault: It Takes All of Us 253

Acknowledgments 257

PROLOGUE

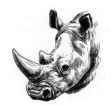

1969, Tierpark Berlin

I shielded my eyes as I stepped out of our taxi into the brilliant sunshine. Despite the fact that we were nearly 4,000 miles from home, the scene we had just left seemed familiar, even comforting. Traffic moved steadily. Pedestrians talked, laughed, and hurried to complete errands. Customers sipped drinks at sidewalk tables in front of Café Adler, the popular coffee shop on the corner.

What lay ahead on *Friedrichstraße*—Friedrich Street—was another matter: barbed wire, concrete barriers, and unsmiling, gray-uniformed border guards carrying submachine guns. It was June 27, 1969, in the midst of the Cold War, and I was 14 years old. My family and I were about to enter Checkpoint Charlie, the infamous crossing station from West Berlin into East Berlin and East Germany. Our little party included my brother, my sister, my mother, and me. The leader of our group was my father, Dr. Kurt Benirschke.

This visit was Dad's idea, of course. Born and raised in Germany, my father was now chair of the department of pathology at Dartmouth's medical school, where he was becoming one of the world's leading authorities on the placenta. Yet he was known for so much more than that. Driven, unconventional, and insatiably curious, Dad was rapidly gaining expertise in reproductive medicine and genetics. He'd discovered that animals could teach us a great deal about abnormalities in human reproduction, which led to his growing passion for studying wildlife and conservation. The day before, we'd visited the Berlin Zoological Garden in West Berlin. Now we were headed to the city's east side and Tierpark Berlin, the largest and most famous animal park behind the Iron Curtain.

In most ways, Dad was fearless. He had a positive, can-do attitude and just expected things to work out. Yet on this day, even my father was anxious. "Remember, no pictures at the checkpoint," he had reminded me and my siblings in the taxi a few minutes before, his tone almost harsh. "No talking, no joking. This is very serious." Only later would I find out that Dad had even more reason to be anxious than I'd realized.

I didn't need the warning. I was already scared down to my tennis shoes. It had been eight years since the Berlin Wall went up practically overnight. Twelve people had died trying to escape East Berlin in the final months of 1961. The next year, 22 people were killed, including 18-year-old Peter Fechter. The teenager was just a few feet east of Checkpoint Charlie, scaling a six-foot-high wall, the final barrier to freedom, when guards shot him in the back and leg and left him to bleed to death on the spot. I was well aware that the men in uniforms weren't carrying weapons for show.

We approached the American side of the checkpoint. It was not much more than a hut with windows, manned by US soldiers. Over the sidewalk to our right was a sign with words printed in block letters: "YOU ARE LEAVING THE AMERICAN SECTOR." Translations in Russian, French, and German appeared lower on the sign. Dad handed our papers to a soldier, and we were cleared to advance.

In single file, with Dad leading the way, we walked silently toward a red-and-white-striped gate and a handful of single-story security structures, all manned by East German *Volkspolizisten*, or "people's police." To my right I noticed steel hedgehog barriers designed to keep tanks and other vehicles from penetrating the East German line of defense in case of attack. The hedgehogs looked like giant versions of jacks from the game I played at home.

I wore shorts and a tennis shirt. A sweater, camera, and change of clothes were tucked into the backpack on my shoulders. I was already sweating, and not just from the heat. I couldn't understand why my parents were both wearing overcoats.

I felt eyes on me as we reached the first security structure. "*Papiere, bitte* [papers, please]," a guard at a window said to Dad. My father handed over our passports. The guard glanced at the documents, raised his head to give Dad an icy stare, and then looked back at the papers.

I realized I wasn't breathing. "What if something is wrong?" I thought. "Will they let us go, or will they throw us in jail? Will they shoot us?"

Finally, the guard handed the papers back to Dad and barked, "*Beeilung* [hurry along]!" We hadn't been detained or searched. We hadn't been shot—at least not yet. I forced myself to take a deep breath.

Still walking single file, we passed more barriers and more border guards. I imagined each man in uniform raising his machine gun and pointing it at our backs after we went by. On the street ahead of us, there was no movement save for the occasional car that had also passed through the checkpoint into East Germany. Compared to West Berlin, we had entered a world that was silent, drab, and potentially deadly.

Once we passed the last of the security checkpoints, Dad grinned. "That went well," he said. I relaxed a little. If Dad was smiling, we must be okay. We'd made it.

Less than an hour later, we were walking the grounds of the 400-acre Tierpark Berlin, founded in 1955 by Heinrich Dathe and famous for, among other things, a visit from Chi-Chi the giant panda a few years earlier. The zoo grounds included Friedrichsfelde Palace, former home of Prussian noble families. As usual, I was fascinated by all the wildlife we walked past.

We soon connected with our four hosts, a group of zoo curators and veterinarians that my dad had met or corresponded with before. They exchanged many smiles and spoke in German. I understood some German, but not enough to follow all of the conversation. At one point, Dad gestured to my brother, Steve; my little sister, Ingrid; and me, and he winked at the men. I wondered what that was about.

We gathered at the zoo restaurant for lunch and more conversation. I noticed Dad and some of the others occasionally glancing sidelong at a man who sat reading in the corner of the room. The man often looked up from his magazine to inspect our group. Later, I was told that he was a zoo supervisor who was suspected of being friendly with the *Stasi*, the East German secret police.

A few minutes later, Dad motioned me over. "Let's visit the restroom," he whispered. "Bring your backpack." The two of us made our way down the hall until we found the right door.

The restroom was deserted. Dad asked me to hand him my backpack. He opened it and rummaged through until he withdrew a small package that was wrapped in brown paper. I didn't even know it was there.

"Dad, what's that?"

My father grinned as he glanced around the room. "It's a present for our friends here," he said. He tucked the package behind the toilet bowl in one of the stalls. "That should do." He pulled another, similar package from the pocket of his overcoat and hid that behind the toilet bowl as well.

"I'll explain later," he said. "For now, please don't ask any more questions about it."

I shrugged my shoulders. Dad was up to something, which wasn't unusual. We returned to the restaurant. He whispered a few words to the veterinarian seated next to him. The man beamed and quietly replied, "*Ich danke dir sehr* [thank you very much]." I wondered what in the world he was so happy about. A few minutes later, the veterinarian excused himself and headed in the direction of the restrooms. He returned shortly after. This scene repeated itself over the course of our meal, only with my parents accompanying my brother and sister to the restrooms. I noticed that Steve and Ingrid both had their backpacks with them. After each bathroom stop, one of our zoo hosts also got up to use the restroom.

When we finished eating, we prepared to see more of the zoo. The staff needed to go back to work, but several made a point of shaking Dad's hand and thanking him before leaving.

It wasn't until we were safely ensconced in our hotel room that evening that Dad explained. The veterinarians at the zoo were desperate to get their hands on M99, a new miracle drug that was far more effective than other methods to anesthetize sick or injured animals. The drug hadn't yet been approved for use in the United States, and certainly no one from the West was authorized by East Germany to deliver it behind the Iron Curtain. But when Dad felt sure he was doing the right thing, he wasn't one to let rules, bureaucracy, or armed East German guards get in his way. He'd hidden significant quantities of the drug, along with all the parts of an immobilization pistol and syringes for delivering the anesthetic, in his and Mom's overcoats and in our backpacks to smuggle them through Checkpoint Charlie. Then, because of concerns that we were being watched by the Stasi, he hid our "presents" in the restroom for the zoo staff to pick up later.

I gulped when I thought about what might have happened if those unfriendly guards had decided to search our belongings. Dad had taken a big risk.

Yet this was Kurt Benirschke: scientist, conservationist, detective, visionary, and daredevil, all rolled into one. He was a man determined to expand his knowledge about the world around him and to use and pass on that knowledge to make the world a better place for humans and wildlife. He would succeed in this quest in ways that he hadn't even imagined yet. Thanks to the discoveries he made and the lives he touched, his legacy is still being written.

My father was a unique man with a unique story—a story that in 1969 was only just beginning.

PART 1
GERMANY

SIGNS AND INCLINATIONS

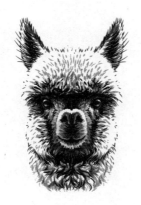

CHAPTER 1

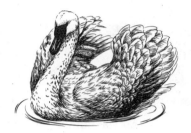

Storm Clouds over Glückstadt

On a cloudy June afternoon in 1934, a 10-year-old boy stood on a grassy patch of land on the east bank of the Lower Elbe River. The boy wore lederhosen, traditional German leather shorts supported by H-shaped suspenders. He had blond hair and a round face, but it was his blue eyes that stood out. They widened with growing interest as he tracked a 200-foot-long freighter gliding slowly along the far bank of the river, past a row of white, red-roofed townhouses.

The boy raced across the grass toward the harbor to get a better look, his long legs covering the ground easily. Soon the ship berthed. The youth watched *Hafenarbeiter* (dock workers) gather to help unload the ship's cargo, which consisted primarily of bundled logs of quebracho wood from Paraguay.

A crane hoisted the quebracho logs a few feet over the river and onto the dock, where the workers waited to haul them away. Suddenly, as one of the bundles was poised over the edge of the freighter, the chain holding them gave way.

"*Achtung* [danger]!" one of the men on the dock yelled.

The logs spilled, some crashing onto the deck of the freighter in a deafening clatter, and more falling between the ship and the dock into the river. Excited by this commotion, the boy watched the logs disappear beneath the surface like torpedoes en route to a target.

The boy wasn't surprised that the logs sank. He knew about quebracho. It was iron-hard and unusually heavy. The logs that didn't end up in the river would be delivered to a nearby factory in Glückstadt, birthplace of naturalist and zoologist Rudolf von Willemoes-Suhm and the town where the boy lived. Tannins were extracted from the trunks for the tanning of cowhides, as Holstein cattle were plentiful in this region of northern Germany. The boy also knew a bit about Paraguay, the subtropical South American country where these trees originated. He wondered what that place was really like—how different it must look from the cultivated fields and river-edge marshes around Glückstadt. He longed to see and experience that exotic land for himself.

The boy had learned geography, and he knew the location of Paraguay because he'd recently taken up stamp collecting. It was the beginning of a lifelong practice of collecting—not just stamps, but anything he decided was interesting and important. At the time, he was fascinated by Paraguay's tiny triangular postage stamps, outdone only by Uruguay's, which were also triangle-shaped and even smaller. He knew about quebracho and the local factory because it sat next to Temming, the paper factory where his father worked. His father had pointed out and explained the function of the quebracho factory to him many times.

This young stamp collector and geography expert was my father, Kurt Benirschke. Born in Glückstadt on May 26, 1924, he was the second child of Friedrich (Fritz) and Marie Benirschke—their only son and spoiled by his mother; older sister, Ilse; and younger sister, Lotte. The family lived in a yellow house at Moltkestraße 8, large for the standards of the time. Dad was an intensely curious, energetic, impatient child who couldn't sit still—there was too much to

CHAPTER 1: STORM CLOUDS OVER GLÜCKSTADT

do. He was also a lackadaisical student. His teachers usually placed him in the front row so they could keep an eye on him when he lost interest in what they were saying and became fidgety.

A child growing up in Glückstadt had plenty to do and explore in the surrounding area. Dad, his sisters, and their friends played ice hockey on a pond behind the house with sticks carved from tree limbs. They also built primitive huts and reenacted adventures of the American Old West from stories they'd read in books by the German writer Karl May. One winter, my dad even floated down the Elbe on an ice floe and had to be rescued by ship.

Dad had just one pet during his childhood, a shepherd dog. But thanks to my grandfather's employer, the family had the use of a large Studebaker, which they drove into the hilly hinterland to see wildlife. Dad often observed deer and partridge on these trips. Seeing beautiful wildlife in their natural habitat made a big impression on his young mind. In those early years, he and his sisters experienced a peaceful, even idyllic youth.

At home, Dad was intrigued by the homemade laboratory my grandfather Fritz had established in the attic of their house. My grandfather cooked soap in large kettles and created ointments and fragrances that he put into gift packages for friends. He also manufactured chartreuse, a pale green liqueur, from brandy and 13 herbs listed in a closely guarded recipe.

Dad was eventually charged with making chartreuse. He became fascinated by the lab equipment as well as the various ingredients he worked with, marveling at how they combined to create an entirely new (and popular) substance. He was also intrigued by an encyclopedia in the attic that showed the anatomy of the human body, with cellophane overlays revealing the different structures.

My grandfather's homemade lab was not just a hobby. Fritz Benirschke was an organic chemist at the paper factory as well as the de facto manager. He'd served as a captain in the Austrian army during World War I before earning his chemistry degree. The position at Temming was the first he found after graduating, a good job in hard times. Unfortunately, he hated Glückstadt. Born in what is now the Czech Republic, my grandfather had trouble adapting to the local language, the food, the lack of "civilization," and the environment. He declared more than once, "This desolate, treeless region must have been created by God in anger!" Although he longed to leave the area and he interviewed for other positions, he would spend the rest of his life in this small town on the Lower Elbe. His frustration at feeling trapped in a place he didn't want to be undoubtedly rubbed off on his son. Dad would always be open to new opportunities and adventures.

Although my grandfather took the family on country drives and other trips, he was not an involved or engaging parent. Other than at the occasional party, he rarely smiled. My dad had a warmer relationship with his mother—my grandmother Marie—who encouraged and took care of him. Dad never got to know his father in a meaningful way. As a teenager, he dented the front left fender of the family car on the night before he was scheduled to take a vacation away from home. He left in the morning without saying anything about the accident. When he returned, he discovered that my grandfather had found out and was furious. Dad was ostracized from the rest of the family, and my grandfather did not speak to him. For weeks, he was forced to eat meals alone in the kitchen, a situation he described as "dreadful." The incident may have made him a more careful driver, but it still didn't slow his enthusiasm for driving fast.

Despite the emotional distance, Dad wanted to emulate his father, who worked incessantly. My grandfather was at Temming day and night, worrying about the operation of the factory, its productivity, and the attitudes of the employees. This tireless dedication was a habit that Dad would incorporate into his own life—and once he was exposed to the lab in the attic, my father decided he wanted to be an organic chemist too.

In 1934, the Benirschkes' tranquil existence was interrupted when my grandfather quit his job at the paper factory over a dispute with the owner about a new manager. A year later, the family moved to a home on Königstraße (King Street) that was owned by my grandmother's family. There, my dad lived in an attic bedroom that overlooked a garden and had a view of the Lower Elbe.

My grandfather Fritz took on his in-laws' coal import and retail business, though not very successfully. Dad accompanied him on trips to the brick factories that sat along the marshes as my grandfather tried to sell anthracite, a high-quality coal imported from England. Then, in 1936, authorities decided to build a navy barracks in Glückstadt. The barracks architect persuaded my grandfather to start a laundry that would serve the townspeople and the navy. He bought a tiny, coal-heated washing machine and a centrifuge, and the family learned how to wash clothes. It was tough going at first, but gradually the business grew. Dad and his younger sister spent most of their "free" time, including weekends, washing, sorting, labeling, packing, and transporting laundry. It was another lesson in the value and necessity of hard work.

Meanwhile, the world around the Benirschke family was rapidly descending into total chaos. At the time the freighter that was filled with quebracho glided into Glückstadt's harbor, Adolf Hitler had already been chancellor of Germany for more than a year. Two months later, Hitler declared himself *Führer*—leader and dictator. His rise to power was swift and merciless. The Nazi Party was decreed the only legal political entity in the nation and was already removing Jews from German society. Intimidation, propaganda, a strengthened economy, and hope for a better future helped Hitler keep the population in line.

In Glückstadt, it was suddenly commonplace to see men in the brownshirt uniforms of the *Sturmabteilung* (Storm Detachment), the Nazi Party's original paramilitary wing. A few teachers and the town mayor were openly pro-Hitler, and some citizens snooped to see if their neighbors were indeed serving

Eintopfessen, the simple stew that the state encouraged families to eat on the first Sunday of the month to save money toward war relief.

In the Benirschke household, however, there was little enthusiasm for the new regime. My grandparents were skeptical of the new leader. My grandmother was against joining the Nazi Party and refused to greet anyone with a "Heil Hitler." My grandfather joined the party out of political necessity but privately remarked that "the big mouth [Hitler] will be our ruin." They listened regularly to BBC radio broadcasts from London to find out what the rest of the world was doing. At the end of the evening, the last person in the room tuned the radio to a German station before turning it off—a safeguard to prevent nosy neighbors from noting any "subversive" influences.

In December 1936, the state decreed mandatory membership in the Hitler Youth, an organization for boys that increasingly took on political and military overtones. Dad was forced to participate in a few camping trips and mock battles, but he hated both the activities and what they stood for, and he never joined the local group. He had already developed a strong sense of what was right and what was wrong that would guide him for the rest of his days.

Soon enough, Adolf Hitler's political and military goals were on display for the world to see. By May 24, 1939, Dad's 15th birthday, the rearmament of Germany was in full swing. Then, on September 1, Nazi Germany invaded Poland. The war was on.

CHAPTER 2

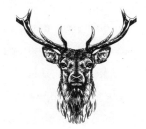

DEATH AND LIFE

War changed everything for Germany, Europe, and eventually the world. Initially, the changes for the Benirschkes were less dramatic. But the family certainly noticed what was going on around them. Dad's small class at school included six boys and six girls when the Nazis overran Poland. Though underage, three of the boys immediately enlisted in the army, and they died at the front. My grandfather forbade my dad from enlisting—not that he had any desire to do so.

Dad was asked to do more and more with the laundry business and matters at home. During the winter, he was responsible for heating up the stoves in every room of the house. In addition, now that there was a risk of enemy bombers at night, he was given "blackout duty"—affixing framed covers to the windows each evening to keep the light from showing.

Even during this uncertain time, Dad was growing up. He had a few romantic relationships with local girls, but he also developed another interest—one that was born out of necessity. In an old wash kitchen at the back of the house, Dad set up a small laboratory. He began experimenting with a variety of chemical compounds under my grandfather's direction.

Because of his background as a chemist, my grandfather was named a chemist in the war effort instead of being drafted into the army. His job was to stay at home and defend citizens from poisonous gases if they were ever deployed. To help, Dad ran the lab and tested material that dropped in the area from enemy planes. It was a chore that he relished. He was a hands-on person, comfortable working with the lab's chemicals and equipment. Even more, the process of discovery was exciting. This practice of testing ideas and uncovering mysteries would energize him for the rest of his life.

In 1942, Dad graduated from the German equivalent of high school. Up to this point, the war had mostly gone Hitler's way, with successful invasions of Poland, Denmark, Norway, France, Belgium, the Netherlands, Greece, and Yugoslavia. But in June 1941, Hitler had launched Operation Barbarossa—the invasion of Russia. It would prove to be a fatal mistake. The initial Nazi advance had been swift, but a bitter winter bogged down its progress. Then, in December 1941, Japan had attacked Pearl Harbor, and the United States entered the war. For those with the vision to see it, the Third Reich was doomed.

My father turned 18 in May 1942, making him eligible for military recruitment. Since he despised the Nazis and what Hitler was doing, he hoped to somehow avoid the draft and continue pursuing his ambition to become an organic chemist. A family friend helped by persuading a physician to declare Kurt Benirschke "physically unfit for duty." Dad was happy to not be going to war, but his excitement was tempered when his sister Ilse's new husband, Kurt Nölke, explained that Dad would have a better chance of getting into the university if he studied medicine, rather than just focused on organic chemistry. After a long discussion with my grandparents, and with their assurances that he could continue to study chemistry after the war was over, Dad agreed to switch his focus to medicine.

He enrolled in the medical school at Hamburg in the fall of 1942 and began to study anatomy, physiology, embryology, organic chemistry, and physics. It opened his eyes to a fascinating new world. Medicine turned out to be far more interesting than he'd anticipated, and he fell in love with all that he was doing. Suddenly, chemistry didn't seem so important.

Then, he received the notice he'd feared. He had been drafted.

Once again, Ilse's husband played a significant role in my father's fate. Kurt Nölke used his connections to get Dad placed on the officer track in the German Air Force. It would give him a chance to continue studying medicine during the war and might allow him to escape the bloodbath at the fronts. Dad got through basic training, and because of his recent medical education, he was assigned to serve as a medic in the air force. In 1943, he was sent to Berlin to continue his medical studies.

Except for a few hours of military training each week, Dad was free to study anatomy as well as observe surgeries and attend lectures on a variety of medical topics. Because so many men were serving in the armed forces, a number of his fellow students were either female—unusual at the time—or amputees who could no longer fight. The students tried to enjoy whatever culture could still be found in Berlin. It was here that my dad developed a lifelong love of opera music. He had been introduced to opera by my grandfather Fritz, who was a violinist as a boy and played chamber music. Dad often attended the opera with his brother-in-law, Kurt Nölke, who was stationed in Berlin.

My dad's reprieve from the military, however, was short-lived. At the end of the semester, during the winter of 1943–44, he was sent to a training ground south of Berlin. For the next four months, in bitter cold, he learned how to fly a glider and how to jump out of airplanes. Paratrooper training was followed by more medical study in the city of Würzburg.

Dad developed a few close friends during this time. One was a fellow medical student and aspiring medic whom he met while in Würzburg. Werner Pagels was from Stralsund on the coast of the Baltic Sea, a German northerner like him. They enjoyed comparing notes about the similarities and differences between growing up in Glückstadt and Stralsund. Unfortunately, Dad learned that Werner was killed in a tank battle just days before the end of the war. He was devastated by the loss of his friend and thought about Werner often over the course of his life.

By mid-1944, Dad had four semesters of medical education under his belt. As far as the military was concerned, he was ready to serve as an air force medic. He was made an officer and sent to an area near the city of Breslau in what is now Poland to support the Nazi war effort against the Soviets. He would be responsible for, among other things, vaccinating troops, caring for the wounded, writing to families of soldiers killed in action, and inspecting pigs to see if they were infected with trichinosis or were safe to eat.

It was a bleak time for proponents of the Nazi regime and not much better for Germans like the Benirschkes who loved their country but opposed Hitler. By the end of 1943, the Nazis had lost nearly all their eastward territorial gains in the Soviet Union. The Allies had landed troops in Sicily and mainland Italy. On June 6, 1944, a massive Allied invasion force struck the beaches of France. Meanwhile, American and British bombers were inflicting heavy damage on both military and civilian targets in Germany. Hitler's grip on Europe was steadily loosening.

That grim summer, Dad was granted a one-week furlough. He was allowed to go home to Glückstadt to see his family and critically ill father. The visit was anything but a vacation.

∞

Dad sat next to a window on the train headed to Glückstadt, hardly believing what he was seeing as the train rumbled across the countryside. Thousands of evacuees filled the roads that ran alongside the train tracks. Old men slowly pushed wheelbarrows filled with all their belongings. Mothers carried their children. Everyone's heads were down as they trudged away from bombed-out houses that would no longer be called home. Many evacuees were from nearby Hamburg, which had been reduced nearly to rubble and was still burning. He wondered where they would go.

Dad still had a home, but he now faced a different kind of loss. His father was dying.

About three years before, one of Lotte's boyfriends, a navy doctor, had observed that my grandfather Fritz, a heavy smoker, was coughing frequently. The doctor had recommended that my grandfather have his larynx examined. At the Hamburg train station following the exam, my grandfather delivered the bad news to his family: he had cancer of the larynx. My grandmother Marie gasped and burst into tears. Dad was too stunned and numb with shock to say anything.

My grandfather had opted for radiation treatment rather than a laryngectomy, but his condition went steadily downhill and soon he was bedridden. With their only son gone to war and no one else available, my grandmother took on leadership of the laundry business as well as caring for her ailing husband. When my grandfather was coherent, he talked of his frustrations and disappointments at Temming but rarely about his family.

When Dad finally arrived at Glückstadt on his furlough, my grandmother greeted him at the family house on Königstraße (King Street) with a warm embrace but sad eyes.

"How is he?" Dad asked after a few moments.

My grandmother shook her head. "Not good," she said. "Not good. The doctor has been giving him morphine."

Dad walked to his father's bedroom, took a deep breath, and entered. He thought he was ready for what he would see, but he was still shocked. His father, once such a strong and energetic man, lay helpless in bed, almost a skeleton. His skin was gray, and a feeding tube ran into his stomach.

My dad swallowed. "Dad," he said, nearly whispering. "Dad, I'm home."

Fritz stirred and groaned, then slowly opened his eyes. For a moment, Dad thought he saw recognition in his father's face. Then my grandfather Fritz grimaced and closed his eyes without saying a word. Despite the morphine, he was clearly in pain and not fully cognizant.

Reluctantly, Dad sat down in a chair next to the bed. My grandfather coughed weakly but did not open his eyes again. Even if they could talk, Dad wondered, what would they say to each other? After a few minutes, he got up and hurried from the room.

The rest of the week passed in a blur. Dad spent most of his time away from the house, visiting friends and avoiding what was going on at home. He couldn't bear the sadness and feeling of helplessness. He hated to watch his father suffer, and their years of emotional disconnection made it that much worse.

On the morning of his last day of furlough, he and my grandmother were in another part of the house while a physician examined my grandfather. When the doctor found them, the look on his face gave it away. "He is at peace now," the doctor said as he bowed his head.

Later that morning, as funeral preparations were being made, Dad was asked to deliver a death notice to the local newspaper. He cried the whole way there, more from guilt over avoiding his father during his last days than from sorrow. He would feel guilty about that week for the rest of his life.

A few days later, he was forced to return to the war.

I asked Dad many times about what it was like to be in a war. Usually, he just shook his head and said, "Rolfie, it's too hard to talk about that. Let's discuss something else." It clearly brought up awful memories and was a subject he never wanted to revisit. It was only from notes he wrote to our family that we have some idea of what he went through.

In early December 1944, Dad was serving with the German Air Force's 1st Parachute Division in the area of Alsace, France, on the Rhine River plain. It was the start of a bitterly cold winter, and the area had been blanketed by heavy snowfall. He would have been dressed in the cornflower blue uniform of the medical corps, complete with an eagle above a swastika on his right breast pocket—though he did not wear it proudly. At least, he told himself, he was attempting to save lives rather than take them.

Though my dad had already seen some combat, he felt the full force of the war in France. American troops were pushing to cross the Rhine River at the town of Haguenau, and the German military's task was to stop them. The two forces met at the small town of Drusenheim, southwest of Haguenau, and fought a particularly fierce battle. Many German troops were wounded or killed, keeping Dad frantically busy during the conflict. He later reported in a diary that it was "terrible" and that he himself "got hit"—although he did not elaborate on his injury.

That night, with no advance notice, the entire division was suddenly loaded onto a train and shipped north. None of them knew where they were going. Their destination turned out to be the southeastern region of the Netherlands, near the Meuse River. Their assignment was to defend the city of Venlo from an American and British offensive.

The Germans and Allies traded bloody raids across the river. Once again, Dad was charged with treating the wounded and writing letters to families of the dead. He was stationed near Nazi V-2 rocket installations that the Allies fiercely bombed and mortared after dark. Terrified, he could barely sleep despite being dog-tired from his long days attending to patients in hospital tents.

One night, in an effort to beat the flea problems that plagued nearly all the soldiers, Dad took refuge in an abandoned house that included an intact bathtub. He poured water into the tub, set a fire underneath to heat the water, stripped, and climbed in. It was an incongruous scene. In the middle of a war zone, he was about to enjoy a few comforts of home: soap and warm water, a private room, a mirror, and a clean towel.

His respite lasted only a few minutes until he heard the unmistakable sound of Allied shells tearing up the countryside. Repeated blows shook the foundation of the house and rocked the water in the tub. As he sat there soaking, the explosions seemed to land ever closer. Feeling unprotected and increasingly alarmed, he jumped out of the tub and dressed hurriedly. He would just have to live with the fleas.

A few nights later, the 1st Parachute Division was on the move again. This time they were headed for what would become known as the Battle of the Bulge. On December 16, Hitler had committed the available troops he had left to launch an all-out offensive intended to stop Allied use of the Belgian port of Antwerp and to split American and British lines. The hope was that it would force the Allies to negotiate a peace treaty in the Axis powers' favor. The push west caught the Allies by surprise and initially was a success for the Nazis. But fierce resistance slowed the German advance on the northern and southern shoulders of the offensive, creating the "bulge" in the center that gave the battle its name. It was then that Allied reinforcements helped turn the tide. The offensive was effectively halted by December 27, even as the battle continued.

The Battle of the Bulge was the longest and bloodiest battle of the war for the United States, and it was also deadly for Germany. Some 100,000 Germans were wounded, captured, killed, or went missing during this campaign. Dad and his companions hid in foxholes in forests as Allied tank shells, mortars, and bombs ripped through snow-covered trees like they were matchsticks. Chunks of shrapnel cut soldiers' bodies in half or ripped off arms or legs, leaving the men screaming for a medic. In the chaos, my father was expected to somehow put the pieces back together. Often the effort was futile.

Of that time, he wrote only, "It was just awful—the confusion, the carnage, the lack of an overall plan or order. It was terrible."

Dad wrote more than once that he feared for his life during the war. Yet he would become a man known for taking chances, for driving fast, for pushing the limits of what was considered acceptable if he thought it was the right thing to do. For my dad, who had confronted the horrors of war and had often looked death in the face, other obstacles and consequences would seem trivial by comparison.

One cold morning in January 1945, Dad woke up to the face of a fellow medic who'd been examining him over the previous few days. He already knew that his skin was yellow and his urine had turned dark brown.

"Good news, my friend," the medic said. "You're lucky. You have acute hepatitis A. You're going home."

That same day, Dad was secured in a stretcher on the front fender of a jeep-style vehicle—his face to the sky so he could watch for Allied fighter-bombers—and driven away from the front to the city of Krefeld. The hospital there was so crowded with badly wounded soldiers that there was no room for an ordinary hepatitis case, so Dad requested and was granted permission to evacuate to his hometown hospital in Glückstadt. When he finally arrived home, his hepatitis symptoms had worsened, and he was in bad shape. My grandmother bathed him to get rid of the fleas. Early the following morning, he was admitted to a navy hospital as he was slipping into a hepatic coma.

For the next week, it was touch and go. Though he had no memory of it, Dad was told that whenever a door slammed, he jumped out of bed, apparently thinking the sound was a grenade.

When he finally began to recover, he learned he would have to return to the western front. Shortly before he was scheduled to be discharged, however, he developed diphtheria. Complications from the treatment kept him in the hospital for weeks more, delaying his return to the front. As Dad recovered from this second illness, he passed the time playing chess with the chief of the navy hospital and dreading what lay ahead.

Then came the stunning report: on April 30, Adolf Hitler had taken his own life in a Berlin bunker. The news was followed on May 8 by Nazi Germany's unconditional surrender to the Allies. The war in Europe was over. Dad's hepatitis had nearly killed him, but that and the diphtheria had kept him away from the deadly fighting at the front—and likely saved his life.

My father debated what to do with his spared life. Like so many other survivors of the war, he would have to pick up the pieces and figure out what would happen next.

CHAPTER 3

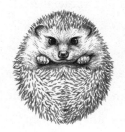

Carpe Diem

I n darkness, a *Kriegslok* (war locomotive) hauled a coal train down the tracks, its engine pistons churning and steam rising from its boiler. An engineer pulled a lever to apply the brakes as the train approached its destination. Farther down the line of cars carrying supplies and fuel, two sooty heads popped out of a mass of black coal. One belonged to my father, Kurt Benirschke. The other belonged to his friend Dr. Steinberger.

The two men were stowaways. Dr. Steinberger hoped to start a medical practice in a town near Munich and wanted to investigate the area. In the weeks after the end of the war, however, railroad transport in Germany was virtually nonexistent except for supply trains. It was also difficult to get clearance to pass from one Allied-occupied zone to another since the Americans, British, and French each controlled different sections of the western half of Germany.

Dad and Dr. Steinberger had decided to risk attempting the 500-mile journey from Glückstadt to Munich on a coal train. Once the train stopped at the station in Munich that night, the two men checked to see if anyone was looking, climbed out of the coal car, lowered themselves to the ground, and slipped into the shadows. They'd made it undetected.

The next morning, Dad and Dr. Steinberger found their way to Mittenwald, the town that would indeed host Dr. Steinberger's new practice and become his home. One of their first stops was a hotel that had been converted into a temporary army hospital for wounded and sick soldiers. As they walked in, Dad noticed the Latin inscription over the door: "*Carpe Diem*," meaning "seize the day." It resonated with him. No one knew what the future held, and no one was guaranteed a future. In the last few months, he'd seen too many lives cut short to think otherwise. Dad decided to make the phrase *carpe diem* his motto for this "next future." There was no time to waste.

Although Dad and the rest of the citizens of Germany were happy that the war was over, they felt despair about what lay ahead. The country was in chaos. No one knew how long the Allied occupation of western Germany would last, what government would be imposed, or how the economy would fare. Refugees from the eastern half of Germany had flooded into the western half to escape the Soviets. Families tried desperately to find out what had happened to sons who had gone missing in action. Food was scarce, often leaving the black market as the only option for obtaining prized goods.

Despite this confusion and turmoil, Dad knew exactly what he wanted to do next. He planned to continue his medical studies back in Hamburg, near his hometown of Glückstadt. The possibilities in medicine continued to intrigue him: there were so many mysteries to solve, so many ways to make a difference in people's lives.

With the war over, Dad was allowed to reenter medical school at the University of Hamburg, and he did so in September 1945. He found and rented a room on the top floor of the Winternitz family's home, which was close to the university hospital and a good arrangement overall. The downside was that he had to endure listening to Mrs. Winternitz, a former opera singer, give lessons to one aspiring student after another in the adjoining room. In addition, it became obvious that the Winternitzes hoped he would take a fancy to their daughter, Daisy, and propose marriage. The family was less than enthusiastic when Dad occasionally invited a different female companion over for tea. Nevertheless, the little room at the top of the Winternitz house would be his primary home for three years.

Dad's main focus was on his studies. At the hospital in Hamburg-Eppendorf, the young medical student attended lectures from 8 a.m. to 5 p.m. every class day, with an hour break for lunch. Among the most captivating subjects for Dad was the course on pathology. Always curious, he frequently stepped into the adjoining autopsy room after lectures to watch students present postmortem findings to a professor. Dad also spent many hours in the obstetrics ward, where he fulfilled the requirement to help deliver babies, and he learned as much as he could about the placenta and the complications that sometimes occurred during childbirth.

Another requirement of his education was a six-month practicum, an unpaid, hands-off work experience in which a student learned by observation. Dad arranged to serve under a local physician, Dr. Heuser, in a typhoid fever hospital near Glückstadt, where an old schoolhouse had been converted into a 72-bed emergency facility. After a few weeks of instruction, Dr. Heuser recognized that my father was especially capable—enough so that the doctor decided to return to his hometown on the Mosel River and leave Dad in charge of the patients and a small staff of nurses. Suddenly, the "hands off" practicum had become hands on.

Even though Dad was eager to take on the challenge, he found it to be difficult work. Because of the severity of typhoid fever and the limited treatments available, about 10 percent of admitted patients died. But the experience was invaluable for his training, and he grew tremendously from the trial-by-fire nature of the work. He also came to appreciate the country lifestyle, the excellent food, and the chance to work with dedicated nurses.

As Dad expanded his medical expertise, he learned humility. One day, a young patient in her third week with a fever developed severe abdominal pain and rigidity, which normally indicated intestinal distress and possibly perforation. Concerned, Dad called for an ambulance and brought his patient to a surgeon in Glückstadt. After a brief examination, the surgeon asked his nurse for a catheter and emptied the patient's bladder. He turned to the young doctor in training and said, "Herr Benirschke, you can take her home again. The 'emergency' you were concerned about was just an overfull bladder." Dad was embarrassed but later admitted it was "a terrific learning experience for me." The amused surgeon told Dad as he was leaving, "You will never make that mistake again."

It was at the typhoid fever hospital that my dad began a lifelong habit. He did the work and initial writing for his first published paper, on malaria, and for his doctoral thesis, on pancreatic involvement in typhoid fever. These efforts would be the first of more than 500 papers he would publish over the next seven decades.

By 1948, his Hamburg studies were complete. He was ready to graduate and earn his medical degree—but only if he could pass the final exams, a brutal, 13-subject series of oral evaluations that took place over six weeks. Dad and the other members of his group began to cram, reading book after book and quizzing each other. Their hard work and commitment paid off: each of them passed every subject. Dad was elated; he couldn't wait to get started in his new career.

He knew that what he needed next was more experience, so he volunteered to work in the bone marrow/leukemia division at the Hamburg hospital. He lived in the hospital basement during his nights on duty and performed hundreds of bone marrow, spleen, and liver biopsies.

After several months at Hamburg, Dad felt he was ready to take the next step in his career. Now he just needed to decide what that step would be. It was a big decision—one that would change the course of his life and involve leaving his country.

In September 1949, my father strode along the wooden platform that extended from the brick passenger station at the busy Hamburg docks. He wore a light gray overcoat, a checkered scarf, and a fedora. He carried a fat suitcase and had 20 English pounds in his pocket. Various family members—including his mother; sisters, Ilse and Lotte; and brother-in-law, Kurt Nölke—trailed behind him. The only son of Fritz and Marie Benirschke had decided that if he was to become the doctor he wanted to be, he would need to leave Germany.

The family was surprised and saddened by Dad's decision, but they came to realize that he had been thinking about it for a while. It had started, in a way, with a tennis date. The previous few summers, Dad and a war buddy named Ulli Firzlaff had lived in a room above a popular tourist restaurant in Hamburg. Dad and Ulli were also unofficial members of a tennis club associated with the restaurant. They couldn't afford the membership, but they were good players and in demand for club tournaments. At a party one evening, Dad met a girl named Reni, which led to a tennis date. They talked about the future and what might happen to each of them as Germany began to rebuild itself after the war.

Reni spoke good English and soon landed a job at the US embassy, but Dad was unsettled. As much as he was enjoying the moment, playing tennis and going out, he knew it was time to make decisions about his future.

My grandmother lobbied for him to take over the family laundry business—and if not that, to at least become a doctor in Glückstadt. But Dad knew he had little aptitude for business. Furthermore, his brother-in-law, Kurt Nölke, seemed perfectly positioned and even eager to take over the laundry. The other option—being a doctor in tiny Glückstadt—appeared equally dreadful to Dad. The last thing he wanted was to end up like his father, trapped in a place he didn't want to be.

My father wanted to pursue a career in medicine, preferably as an academic.

He felt this was where he could make a difference. As a professor, he could guide and instruct students, and he would have the freedom to explore his own medical interests.

At the time, everything in Germany was uncertain. Dad toyed with the idea of staying for a while, thinking conditions might improve and he could have a successful career in Germany. But things were too unsettled, and he ultimately decided he did not want to wait. He was certain that the best opportunities to learn and advance would be found elsewhere, a belief he often conveyed to Reni.

Out of the blue one Sunday, Reni called and told Dad that the next morning, the US consulate was registering candidates for possible immigration to America. At Reni's urging, he got up early the next morning and joined hundreds of other German citizens hoping for a chance at a new start. He eagerly stood in line with them for the next four hours, waiting for a "golden ticket" card with a registration number. The crowd had been told that only 50 people from northern Germany would be allowed to immigrate to the United States that year, so the chances were slim for everyone. When Dad finally received his card, however, he was devastated: his number was 740. He had no chance. It was over. Done. He was stuck in Germany, and there was nothing he could do about it.

Reni saw how crushed Dad was. She knew how much he'd been looking forward to leaving Germany and starting his medical career.

"Kurt, quickly, give me your number," she said. Confused, he handed Reni the card, and she disappeared into the consulate office where she worked. A few minutes later, she came out and gave his number back—only it wasn't the same number. Reni had found a way to eliminate the "7" from his card. Suddenly, Dad was candidate number 40, and he was going to America after all. He was stunned, overwhelmed, and so grateful to Reni. The stoic young man who had been through so much, seen such pain and suffering during the war, was now suddenly overcome with emotion. He began sobbing uncontrollably. Reni knew she was losing a friend but couldn't have been happier for him. In the decades that followed, my father would speak of this moment often; he considered it the single biggest break of his life.

Dad knew little about the United States except that it had just helped destroy his native country. He spoke no English. His teachers had provided virtually no information on US history, and because everyone in Germany had considered America the enemy during the war, he was more than a little uneasy at the prospect of going there.

As he stood on the Hamburg dock a few days later, suitcase in hand, and prepared to board a small freighter, the significance of what he was about to do began to sink in. He had strong, mixed emotions as he leaned over to hug and kiss his mother, sisters, and Reni. When would he see them all next? *Would* he see them again? Could he survive on his own?

Then my father gathered himself and straightened to his full six feet. Yes. This was the right choice. He was 25 years old, had survived a devastating war, and had worked diligently to earn a degree in medicine, a field he loved. It was time to make his mark on the world. *Carpe diem.* He walked up the gangplank to the freighter without looking back. He was on his way.

PART 2
BOSTON

A Growing Brood

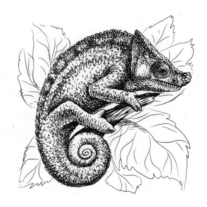

CHAPTER 4

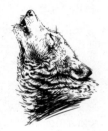

MAKING A START

Although Kurt Benirschke landed in America with little more than a suitcase and a dictionary, he arrived with one much more important asset—an expectation that he would succeed. His family thought differently, anticipating he'd be back in Germany within six months. Despite their lack of faith, he truly believed that he could do anything if he put his mind to it and that things would work out.

His first challenge was learning to speak a new language. To help with that, my grandmother arranged for him to spend the first month of his journey in London with the Jevons family. Dad had met John Jevons the previous Christmas in Glückstadt, where John had been stationed with the British Army. They were about the same age and shared a love of music. They had even played Beethoven sonatas together, John on violin and Dad on piano. In London, John showed him around the city, taking him to museums, hospitals, and symphony performances at the Royal Albert Hall. All the while, Dad referred to his little dictionary and pestered John with questions about how to say things in English.

When Dad's time in London was up, he thanked his friend and boarded the SS *Sacramento* for the three-week journey across the Atlantic Ocean to New York. While on board, he continued to try to advance his language skills. He met an artist from New York, Mrs. Bethers, who was willing to help him with his pronunciation. They spent hours walking up and down the deck together, even during rainstorms, while Dad practiced his "th" sounds and other tricky parts of the English language.

Finally, the skyscrapers of New York City came into view. Dad felt a tingle in his soul as he took it all in, wondering what lay ahead. He had finally arrived at his new home and was determined to make the most of it. After clearing the immigration process, his "guarantor" (sponsor), J. J. Augustin, picked him up at the dock. Originally from Glückstadt, J. J. had moved to America several years before and now worked as a publishing house representative. For the first time in two months, Dad was able to speak his native language and know he was being understood. It was a relief.

He roomed with J. J. on Long Island and got a job with J. J.'s publishing house, where he delivered books and ran errands. He continued to learn English by listening to people on the subway and talking with his barber and work contacts. He also convinced a former schoolteacher near Columbia University to give him private lessons. Every day, he became more proficient.

Meanwhile, Dad worked on finding and securing a medical internship. Every Thursday, he visited the library at Columbia's medical center to look for internship openings in the latest issue of the *Journal of the American Medical Association*. He found many listings, but most were for positions in faraway cities like Miami, Toledo, or Chicago. Dad hardly knew where those places were, but after checking on a map, he realized he couldn't afford the cost of getting to the interview anyway. Undeterred, he kept looking.

It was on an errand for the publishing house one morning that Dad thought his fortunes might have changed. He had just passed a building with a huge brass plaque over the entrance that read, "Office for the Placement of Displaced Physicians." "Well, that's for me," Dad thought, so he went inside to check it out. After speaking with someone at the front desk, he decided to fill out a form and register. Ultimately, that didn't lead to anything, because he never heard back from the organization. But in a moment of serendipity, what happened while he was in the building changed his life.

Dad was in the hallway outside the office, preparing to leave, when he overheard a man tell someone in German that there was an internship available in Teaneck, New Jersey. He could hardly believe what he was hearing.

"Teaneck," he thought. "I've seen the bus signs to Teaneck right by Columbia's medical center. I think I can find that place."

Equipped with this new lead, my dad learned that the internship committee at Holy Name Medical Center in Teaneck met every Thursday at 5 p.m. On the following Thursday, he made his way by bus and stood before a group of physicians, answering questions about his qualifications and experience. One of the interviewers spoke German and translated the conversation for the others.

After a few minutes of this awkward exchange, Dad interrupted the translator. "I can save us all some time," he said. "You don't have to translate for me. I understand and can speak some English."

The committee members exchanged glances. One member nodded to another, who then addressed my father. "If you can speak English, you're hired."

And that was it. Dad began work as an intern for Holy Name Medical Center on January 1, 1950, earning $100 a month plus room and board.

∞

For the next year and a half, Dad received well-rounded training in Teaneck, New Jersey, rotating from one specialty to another. His first assignment was to assist a surgeon on a patient with breast cancer. After the surgery rotation came a focus on general medicine, pediatrics, obstetrics, radiology, the outpatient department, and pathology. Some of the rotations lasted as long as three months. Dad took it all in, loving every minute he was in the hospital.

The idea of America as a melting pot was certainly evident at Holy Name Medical Center. All the other interns, it seemed, were first- or second-generation immigrants. One was from Italy, another from Russia, two were Irish, and two were from Estonia. The latter two spoke German, which made Dad feel even more at home. Minerva, the hospital diener (a morgue worker responsible for handling bodies), was Estonian and spoke German. She cleaned the interns' rooms and looked after the newcomers in addition to working as a morgue attendant and autopsy technician.

Unfortunately, most of the doctors and nurses at Holy Name did not go to great lengths to educate their interns. A few gave lectures, but the lectures were rare and not especially helpful. Dad learned the most from his own experiences, from comparing notes with his fellow interns, and from watching how others did things.

One of the things he noticed was that Dr. Luther Markley, the Holy Name pathologist, often drove to New York City to visit another pathologist. When Dad asked what the doctor was doing, he found out that Dr. Markley was sending bone marrow slides to be interpreted. Dr. Markley had never been trained in how to read the slides. Sensing an opportunity, Dad offered to help, having had quite a bit of experience doing bone marrow interpretations in Hamburg after the war. His offer was gratefully accepted, and he found himself working part-time for the pathology department.

Dr. Markley took a liking to this bright young intern. Their friendship grew, and soon the doctor was loaning his gray 1948 Oldsmobile to Dad so he could make house calls to start IVs for transfusions to patients with aplastic anemia. One day, he noticed Dr. Markley's paycheck sitting on the front seat of the Oldsmobile. Dad couldn't resist peeking. He was stunned to learn that the doctor's annual salary was a whopping $30,000!

But the job was never about money for Dad. He loved learning about pathology, and his role in the department expanded. He began performing autopsies and assisting with surgeries. He studied the science behind all kinds of diseases, why things went wrong, and how disease affected different systems in the body. Dr. Markley recognized his interest and suggested that with all the experience he was gaining, he should make pathology his career.

Since Dad's Holy Name internship would end on June 30, 1951, Dr. Markley offered to arrange a pathology residency for him in New York City so he could continue his studies. Dad was grateful. Dr. Markley had given him the chance to discover a passion for pathology. Equally important, he had demonstrated how a good mentor could influence a student, a lesson that Dad would remember.

My father's medical career was starting to take shape, but his romantic life was more in flux. Although his English was improving rapidly, it was certainly easier to communicate with young women who spoke his native tongue. Dad had taken a fancy to Hilja, one of the two German-speaking interns at Holy Name. But Hilja seemed to have little interest in the aspiring pathologist from Glückstadt and hardly gave him the time of day.

One morning, Dad entered the solarium to give an injection to a patient and spotted a new nurse at the desk—my mother. She was a brunette who had a dimple in her left cheek and a beautiful smile. He heard her speaking in German to one of the other nurses. Not wanting to miss the opportunity, Dad mustered his courage and introduced himself. She said her name was Marion Waldhausen.

They exchanged a few words. Before the conversation was over, Dad somehow managed to squirt her with a syringe of saline solution that he'd been holding. He never explained whether this was by accident or on purpose, but it had its effect: my mom, Marion, didn't forget that first meeting.

He continued to run into the new nurse at the hospital, and they sometimes attended to patients together. Dad was very good at starting IVs but not very good at asking for a date. Eventually, he got up the nerve and asked her out to dinner.

Marion Waldhausen was born in the United States and spent most of her formative years in Englewood, New Jersey. Her German father, Max, was the principal New York representative of the Siemens corporation, which was founded in Germany and manufactured medical equipment, among other products. When World War II broke out, the family returned to Germany to escape internment in the United States. However, Allied bombs had destroyed their house in Berlin. After the war, the US consulate in Germany pressured Mom to return to the United States, hinting that her US citizenship could be revoked if she didn't. In January 1947, she traveled with her mother, Agnes, and younger brother, John, by train through war-ravaged Germany to the port at Bremerhaven. As her brother John later wrote, "For Marion this was a tough moment, to go to America at age 19, alone. But Marion did not hesitate and went without complaint or overt fear, characteristics that she had always shown."

She settled in New Jersey with family friends and entered a nursing program that placed her at Holy Name. Since she had attended the German equivalent of high school but had never finished, she also took night classes to earn an American diploma.

With such similar backgrounds and experiences, my parents became friends and enjoyed going out to dinner or a movie whenever they could. They got to know each other best at the hospital, though. Mom called Dad at all hours and asked for help with giving injections or starting IVs in elderly ladies or others whose veins were difficult to find. He was, of course, happy to comply.

Despite the promising start with Mom, Dad couldn't quite get Hilja off his mind. One night, he and Mom went dancing at the Ambassador Hotel in New York City, where they had a great time. At the end of the evening, they were awarded a bottle of champagne. Unfortunately, Dad later made the mistake of drinking that bottle with Hilja on her birthday, much to Mom's irritation.

It seemed that my father needed a nudge to clear his muddled thinking. Once again, fate would step in. It was Dr. Markley who would provide much-needed wisdom and again alter the trajectory of Dad's personal life and his career.

"I know you're planning on going to New York when your internship ends," Dr. Markley told Dad one morning in early 1951. "But would you like to do something even better? Harvard has just hired a new pathology department chairman, and he's looking for interns."

Dad didn't know where Harvard was or even how to spell it. But Dr. Markley explained the institution's reputation for quality. His persuasive description made Dad want to check it out and learn more. Dr. Markley helped him arrange an interview with Clinton "Bud" Hawn, Harvard's newly named pathologist. At the time, Dr. Hawn was still with a hospital in Cooperstown in upstate New York. The interview was set for 8 a.m. on a Saturday in March.

On the Friday before the interview, Dad had rented a car and was about to leave the hospital when he saw my mom just getting off her shift. On impulse, he explained his plans and asked if she was interested in joining him for the trip. To his surprise, she said yes. After a stop for a change of clothes, they were off.

The trip included a visit with friends in Poughkeepsie and driving through a snowstorm, but they made it to Cooperstown in time for the interview. It was still snowing in the picturesque community when they arrived. Dad got out of the car for his interview, while Mom snuggled into the backseat to catch up on sleep.

Dad's conversation with Dr. Hawn went well. To my father's surprise, Hawn offered him one of three Harvard pathology residency positions at Peter Bent Brigham Hospital (now Brigham and Women's Hospital) in Boston. Ecstatic, Dad immediately accepted. Then Dr. Hawn invited him to lunch to formally welcome him to the team. Dad was excited to join the team for lunch, but first he had to explain to his new boss that he had a "friend" waiting in the car. He was embarrassed to add that the friend was a "she." Dr. Hawn couldn't believe that his new resident had kept a young woman waiting in a freezing car for hours. They made their way to the parking lot to get my still-sleeping mother.

Mom, who was not fully awake and was unaware that Dad was with someone, asked within earshot of Dr. Hawn, "Was he nice?" Dad felt even more embarrassed. However, the doctor was charmed by the whole incident, and the trio went inside to enjoy a celebratory lunch. It was, my father later wrote, "a most successful and lovely weekend"—and the beginning of much, much more.

CHAPTER 5

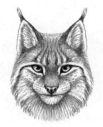

Grand Rounds ... and Rings

On Dad's first night of work, he quickly learned that life at Peter Bent Brigham Hospital in Boston would be very different from what he'd experienced in Teaneck, New Jersey. Expectations were much higher here—but so was the level of cooperation and training.

Dad had met his new roommate, fellow pathology resident and Lebanon native Najib Abu-Haydar, the evening before. They were both excited to start their training. The next day, they were given their first assignment: to perform a frozen section biopsy to determine if a patient's brain tumor was benign or malignant. Unfortunately, neither of them knew exactly how to perform the procedure. They were wondering how to proceed when neurosurgeon Don Matson rescued the fledgling residents. He said that if Dad and Najib would open the pathology lab, he would demonstrate the procedure. The three men became good friends that night.

It was a sign of things to come, in both education and collegiality. Dad and Najib loved it. Every Thursday morning, they went to "Grand Rounds," a four-hour teaching and review session that was attended by staff and other physicians who wanted to learn. Cases were discussed in great detail, adding depth to their medical knowledge. New medicine was being discovered or invented at "the Brigham," as people called it, almost every day.

Over the next year, Dad, Najib, and a third pathology resident, Jim McAdams, performed some 250 autopsies and 5,000 minor or major surgeries. They were frequently called on to present findings after these procedures, which led to more valuable learning. Through a potent mix of good fortune, foresight, and hard work, my father, Kurt Benirschke, had found himself at ground zero for some of the most interesting and exciting developments in the medical world.

In 1951, the same year that Dad started at the Brigham, Dr. Joseph Murray returned to the surgical staff. Murray had developed an interest in transplantation while caring for wounded American soldiers during World War II. Dad joined Dr. Murray, Brigham surgeon John Merrill, and the hospital's chief resident in surgery, David Hume, on annual trips to the New York Academy of Medicine to hear the nation's leading experts discuss transplant immunology.

The process of transplanting kidneys was in its infancy at the time. In fact, Dad had performed many autopsies on patients who'd received healthy kidneys, only to see the kidneys fail. In 1954, at Peter Bent Brigham Hospital, Murray—assisted by Merrill, Hume, and others—would perform the world's first successful human kidney transplant. The patient, Richard Herrick, would live another eight years after receiving a healthy kidney from his twin brother, Ronald. Murray would eventually earn a Nobel Prize for this and other contributions to organ and cell transplantation.

Meanwhile, other medical advances were taking place at the hospital. Dad was assisting Dr. Don Matson with a relatively new treatment for breast cancer, which involved removing the pituitary gland. Another leading research scientist at the Brigham, cardiologist Dwight Harken, was refining his new technique for correcting the narrowing of a patient's mitral heart valve. Dr. Harken was also credited with introducing the concept of the hospital's intensive care unit.

In addition, George Thorn, the Brigham's chief of medicine, was beginning breakthrough studies investigating the connection between cortisol and stress. He pioneered the use of cortisone as a treatment for Addison's disease, and his research led to new treatments for diseases such as hypertension, rheumatoid arthritis, and diabetes. Dr. Hume, who was working with Thorn, wanted to know more about promising German research in this area but couldn't read the papers. Dad supplemented his $42.50-per-month income by translating the articles into English at $5 an hour. More important to him than the money was the knowledge he was gaining in the process.

Dad was fortunate to be working with some of the brightest minds in medicine, and the highly charged atmosphere was a heady tonic for him. He also enjoyed and benefited from the family culture at the Brigham. Every evening, a handful of residents and interns gathered in the hospital cafeteria to eat the leftovers from patients' meals as their dinner and talk about medicine, politics, and whatever else came to mind. He made several lifelong friends there who collaborated, pushed each other in their medical studies, and celebrated each other's successes.

Dad's medical experience and knowledge were advancing at a rapid rate. Soon the same would also be said about his romantic life.

In the fall of 1951, my father drove to Teaneck for a weekend visit. He'd been at Holy Name Medical Center only a short time when an intern casually said, "You should check in on Miss Waldhausen. She's just been operated on for a large kidney stone, and she might like to see you again." The operation was news to Dad. He located the room and found her recovering in bed. Her own mother, Agnes, sat at her side.

My mom, Marion, had been shopping in New York and developed severe pain in her side, which led to the discovery of the large stone and the need for surgery. An exam revealed that she now had kidney stones on her other side as well, which required a second surgery at Holy Name.

Dad was convinced that she would receive much better care at the Brigham—as well as more personal attention from a certain resident pathologist. "You don't need to have the operation here," he said. "I can arrange for you to come to the Brigham in Boston. Then we can figure out what's causing these stones when we take them out."

Thanks to a little persuasion from Dad, George Thorn included Mom in his study of patients with hyperparathyroidism, and the plan was set. The surgery and monthlong recovery in Boston gave my parents more time to get reacquainted. It also gave another Brigham intern time to fall in love with my mother, leaving Dad quite jealous. Mom was really more interested in her solicitous caretaker from Glückstadt, but she wasn't above letting Dad know that she had another suitor.

There was an additional obstacle to my dad's growing affection for my mom. My maternal grandmother, Agnes, who had settled in Great Falls, Montana, wanted Mom to join her. Mom agreed to move there shortly after her discharge from the hospital and continue her nursing career in Montana after she recovered. When Dad got word of this, he felt mounting pressure to do something. He was worried that if he didn't, he might never see my mother again.

On the day of her discharge, Mom's travel arrangements to Montana had already been made. That morning, Bud Hawn called Dad into his office. Dr. Hawn seemed just as agitated now as he'd been months earlier when he learned that Dad had left Mom in the car during their first meeting.

Hawn wasted no time getting to the point. "Kurt, you're a complete fool," he said. "Do you really want to let that girl escape to the Wild West, never to see her again? You'll never find another one like her in your life. You're crazy if you don't marry her."

Dad shook his head. "I can't," he said. "I can't marry someone when I'm making less than 45 bucks a month. How could I support her? I still have more training to do. It's not likely I'll be making much more anytime soon."

Later that day, Dad sadly said goodbye to Mom. But even as he did, he couldn't get Dr. Hawn's admonition out of his mind. Despite his meager salary, maybe there was a way to make it work. Dad believed Marion Waldhausen *was* a once-in-a-lifetime girl, and they were so good together. Could they—should they—get married after all?

Mom did leave for Great Falls. But their relationship continued via a series of long letters that flew back and forth, and it soon became clear to my parents that they were meant for each other. As to who proposed marriage first—that was their secret. But since Dad later admitted to making Mom destroy the letters "so that the truth could never be found out," it's not hard to guess what happened. In any event, they were engaged by spring 1952, with the wedding planned for just a few weeks later, on May 17.

There was more drama ahead when it came time for Dad to drive west for the wedding. His 1947 Nash needed significant repairs before it could make the trip to Montana, and he had already spent the few dollars he'd managed to save. Dad went to the only place he could think of, the office of the Brigham's administrator, to plead for a loan. The administrator, Ms. Chase, had taken a liking to the hardworking young resident. She pulled out a large roll of bills and handed my father $500 in cash. "Pay me back when you can," she said with a smile. "Now go marry that beauty!"

Several days later, on a Friday night, Dad got off work and began the long trek to Montana. Accompanied only by what he called "awful" country music playing on a tape deck, he made few stops and was awed by the size of his adopted country. He arrived in Great Falls on Tuesday afternoon, just four days before the wedding. When he drove to my mother's house and discovered she was out, he decided to find the nearest bar for a meal and a beer. The barkeeper must have been surprised. The long-legged stranger from Boston had traveled in lederhosen—a little different from the jeans and cowboy boots worn by most of the patrons.

The wedding, at a Catholic church in Great Falls, was a success. Family friends provided Mom with a wedding dress, organized a reception dinner, and gave the couple many practical gifts. They also added to the festive atmosphere by tying beer cans to the bumper of Dad's freshly washed Nash, an American tradition. The newlyweds spent the night at a nearby resort, loaded the car the next day, and headed off to Boston to start their new life together.

But it wasn't to be a smooth ride.

My parents were on a Wyoming highway when they heard a terrible grinding noise emanating from the Nash's engine. They turned off at the next exit and limped into a small town, looking for help. They eventually found a mechanic who identified the problem: a large bearing had burned out, and with it, the front and rear gears. The fix wouldn't be cheap. Unfortunately, most of the $500 that Dad had borrowed was already gone, and he didn't have enough left for the repairs. A call for help to J. J. Augustin, his former roommate and benefactor in New York, did not go as expected. J. J.'s reply was, "You got yourself into this mess, so get yourself out."

Desperate and seemingly without options, Dad tried offering Mom's engagement and wedding rings as payment to the mechanic. Given that the couple had been married only a few days, it was a good thing that the mechanic turned him down. After calling everyone he could think of who might help, Dad finally reached a pathologist that he'd befriended in Great Falls. The man agreed to wire a $200 loan to bail out the young couple.

They were back on the road again, but due to the unexpected stay in Wyoming, they had to rush back to Boston so Dad could report for work on time. While driving through West Virginia, he asked his new wife for a kiss. Whether it was lack of sleep, his fast driving, the offer to trade her rings, or that he "was unshaven" (as she stated), Mom refused. Her rebuffed husband jokingly pretended to throw his wedding ring out the window of the speeding car. At that moment, the Nash hit a bump in the road and the ring really did go flying.

Horrified, Mom insisted that Dad stop the car immediately, walk back to the spot, and find the ring. The man who would one day be lauded as a world leader in medicine and wildlife conservation was on his hands and knees in the grass next to the highway, looking for his ring as cars whizzed past. By some miracle, he found it, which may have saved his new marriage—if not his pride.

Despite the bumps in the road, the Benirschkes made it back to Boston, still speaking to each other and still in possession of their rings. They were frazzled and in debt, but they were together. They didn't know it at the time, but theirs was a partnership that would endure for 66 adventurous years.

CHAPTER 6

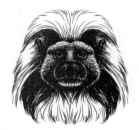

Little Zoo on Bird Hill

K urt and Marion Benirschke lay on the floor in the dark, trying to fall asleep. Loud talk, clinking glasses, and jukebox music drifted up through the floorboards of their tiny one-room apartment, which was perched directly above the Lobster Claw, a bar in downtown Boston. The newlyweds had no furniture and used discarded orange crates as chairs and a table. Only later did they acquire such luxuries as a mattress, a secondhand Persian rug to cover the floor and dampen the sounds from the bar, and a refrigerator that ran constantly to keep its contents "luke-cold."

With my dad just starting his career, my mom's salary was important. Because of the money they owed after the wedding and their expensive trip home, Mom signed on as a nurse at Peter Bent Brigham Hospital. Dad worked long hours, and he supplemented their income by donating blood every month and performing autopsies for a commercial laboratory in the evenings. Mom often accompanied him. Besides dealing with tight finances, she was learning to cook to Dad's often-picky taste. On special occasions, she prepared favorites from his mother's home-cooking recipe book: goose, flounder, asparagus, and white spring potatoes.

Despite their early challenges, my parents were happy and determined to make the most of their new life. Dad was doing important work he loved with talented colleagues he respected. It was the kind of life he'd dreamed of, and now he had a partner to share it. Mom loved her work as a nurse, and she had found a partner with a bright future who was a companion and a confidante—someone who would help her raise a family.

Dad had a favorite story from that time. One night, when my parents were driving on Route 1 toward Providence, Rhode Island, for one of my father's commercial lab autopsies, they rounded a bend and saw a huge billboard announcing, "Greyhound Races Tonight at 8 p.m." Mom exclaimed, "Wow, I didn't know they raced buses!" Dad loved telling that story because it recalled an innocent and carefree time for both of them.

That summer he started the next phase of his Harvard residency at Boston Lying-In Hospital, so named because it was originally established for low-income women who needed a place to "lie in" and recover after delivering a baby. His salary improved to $100 a month. Since he didn't have to pay for his hospital cafeteria meals, he loaded up his tray and shared his food with Mom, who now worked at the Lying-In Hospital as well.

They soon discovered that they needed to look for more creative ways to save money. Early in 1953, Mom revealed that she was pregnant. The news was a bit of a shock to Dad, who wanted kids but hadn't given the matter much thought. Nevertheless, two Benirschkes were about to become three.

The pregnancy proceeded smoothly through the spring and summer. Mom worked as a nurse until she was physically unable to continue. Then, on August 16, my older brother, Stephen Kurt Benirschke, entered the world. My parents were proud and pleased, although a bit overwhelmed by the new responsibility.

CHAPTER 6: LITTLE ZOO ON BIRD HILL

Unfortunately, the happy news was tempered by a loss. Earlier that summer, Dad's mother—my grandmother Marie—had finally been able to make the long trip from Glückstadt to Boston to visit. She enjoyed meeting Mom and seeing her son for the first time in four years. Since my parents barely had room for themselves in their tiny apartment, they arranged for her to take the bus to Montana so she could see the country and stay for a few weeks with Mom's mother, my grandmother Agnes. Marie enjoyed the trip and returned after Steve's birth to meet her new grandson before traveling back to Germany. Not long after her return home, however, she went to the hospital for a gallbladder operation. Shortly after the surgery, she got out of bed, had a massive pulmonary embolism, and died. Dad was devastated, but he couldn't afford to go home for the funeral. He was grateful his mother had been able to see her new grandson, but he wished he'd spent more time with her during her visit. Once again, he was left feeling guilty after the death of a parent.

Baby Steve's first quarters consisted of a crib in the bathroom of my parents' one-room apartment. The Benirschkes needed a bigger place to live. On one of her neighborhood walks, Mom discovered an apartment complex that was being rebuilt on Francis Street. The units had two bedrooms, a small bathroom, and a kitchen nook, and the building was so close to Dad's work that he could walk home for lunch.

As soon as an apartment was available, they moved in. Mom worked to make the apartment a home while Dad continued to perform commercial autopsies and translate articles from German to English to earn extra money for the rent. He also learned to change diapers, studied for the test that would make him a US citizen, and took up photography, often spreading out the developed film on an ironing board in the evenings. His seemingly endless supply of energy was remarkable, and it was a good thing, because he would need even more.

Mom was pregnant again, this time with me, Rolf Joachim Benirschke. I was born on February 7, 1955, and my younger sister, Ingrid Marie Benirschke, followed on April 16, 1956. The next year, our expanded family moved into a house with a big yard on Bird Hill Avenue in the town of Wellesley, a suburb of Boston. Dad learned how to mow grass, built a darkroom in the cellar, and enjoyed having a place where his family could grow.

His career was thriving as well. He added more residencies to his résumé, including the Free Hospital for Women and Boston Children's Hospital. In 1954, as part of his Harvard residency, he was promoted to assistant pathologist at both the Brigham and Boston Lying-In hospitals. His residency, however, was nearly up. Where would he go next?

Dad had a plan. As he told a friend, "My goal is to someday become chief pathologist at the Lying-In Hospital." He was soon named chief resident at the Lying-In, Harvard's second-largest teaching hospital. Then Don McKay, the hospital's chief pathologist, was drafted to serve in the Korean War. McKay's replacement stayed only a short time before taking a position in New York, and it seemed Dad's hopes were about to come true.

But his goal would not be realized quite that easily. His temporary, five-year license for practicing medicine in Massachusetts was about to expire, and "foreigners" were prohibited from applying for a permanent license. A colleague tried to get Dad inducted into the Massachusetts Medical Society, thinking that would solve the issue, but his application was voted down. The next morning, a Boston newspaper article with the headline, "German-educated pathologist blackballed by Massachusetts Medical Society" condemned the state's medical licensure system. A week later, the chastised authorities "invited" Dad to sit for the licensure examination. Even though he had no time to prepare, he passed the three-day exam. Shortly after, he was officially named pathologist in chief at the Boston Lying-In Hospital. It was, he would write, "a dream fulfilled."

CHAPTER 6: LITTLE ZOO ON BIRD HILL

My father was fascinated by pathology, but it was during his residency years that he developed the specific interests that dominated the rest of his career. One of the moments that inspired these passions was a comment my mother made one evening before Steve was born.

Among the many mysteries that Dad pondered was why babies with anencephaly—born without parts of the brain and skull—had unusually small adrenal glands. Since my parents couldn't afford much in the way of entertainment, they began spending evenings at the Boston Lying-In, looking up past cases of anencephaly. On one of those evenings, Mom set down the paper she was holding and looked at Dad. "You know," she said, "it's amazing that in many of these cases the baby has only a single umbilical artery."

Dad sat back in his chair. "Isn't that interesting?" he said. "I wonder why." Already his mind was searching for answers. "Somebody," he said after another moment, "ought to start looking at all their placentas and see if they can learn something."

In 1953, the placenta was in many ways a mystery, referred to as the "afterbirth" and regarded by the majority of medical professionals as an afterthought. At birth, the placenta averaged about nine inches in length, weighed just over a pound, and was dark red-blue or crimson in color. Doctors understood that the placenta developed during pregnancy and attached to the wall of the uterus, and that blood filtering oxygen and other important nutrients passed from the placenta to the growing baby via the umbilical cord. The medical community also understood that placental problems could develop during pregnancy. The placenta might separate from the uterus before delivery (placental abruption), shift to block the cervix (placenta previa), or remain attached to the uterine wall after childbirth (placenta accrete). Despite these risk factors, it seemed that no one had pursued placental pathology seriously.

Dad began to realize from numerous post-birth examinations how often the placenta provided clues to what had gone wrong with a pregnancy and what those clues might predict about the mother and baby. For example, an analysis might reveal that a stillbirth had been caused by an infection in the placenta. A closer look at the placenta might also uncover the presence of previously undetected diseases or infections in the baby or mother and provide insight about how to treat a mother's future pregnancies. The placenta might even predict a child's long-term health.

Mom's observation, combined with the promise of those potential discoveries, proved irresistible to Dad. He asked for and was granted permission by the authorities at the Boston Lying-In and other regional hospitals to examine every placenta delivered over the next year—about 5,000 of them! He found that about 1 percent of the placentas had a single umbilical artery, and that congenital abnormalities and deaths were more common in those cases.

Naturally, Dad wrote a paper on the results, but he didn't stop there. Questions danced in his mind. How did the placenta develop, and how exactly did its development influence fetal growth and health? Were all placentas similar in function? What was their transport and endocrine function? Was there a connection between the placenta and premature birth, or the placenta and resulting death? Dad needed to know more. He would become so immersed in this work and so knowledgeable over the course of his career that he was often introduced as the "world's leading authority on the placenta."

His curiosity extended to many other perinatal issues (challenges and abnormalities immediately before and after birth). Dad was particularly intrigued by twins and the medical challenges surrounding their birth, including the fact that twin babies died much more frequently than single babies.

Dad's interest in twin births had been piqued when Mom was pregnant with Steve. At that time, he learned that a patient at the hospital named Mrs. Page was pregnant with fetuses that had twin-twin transfusion syndrome, meaning one fetus was receiving more blood than the other. Dad was able to follow Mrs. Page's progress closely because Mom was seeing the same doctor in the same hospital. Sadly, one of the Page twins died and was flattened between the other fetus and the mother's uterine wall, a rare condition known as fetus papyraceus. At the time, little was known about the causes and appropriate treatments for this unusual phenomenon. When Mom and Mrs. Page went into labor at nearly the same time at the hospital, Dad couldn't tear himself away from the fascinating problem pregnancy. In fact, he ended up missing the birth of his first child—something Mom was not happy about, although she grew to accept it in time.

Dad's curiosity would make him an expert on perinatal issues not just for humans, but eventually the animal world too. His interest began with a unique animal called a nine-banded armadillo. This armored, nocturnal insectivore is the most common of the armadillos and makes its home mostly in the southern United States and in Central and South America. The nine-banded armadillo *always* produces quadruplets—four identical embryos attached to a common placenta. My dad realized these quadruplets were almost always free of the complications that could be found in human twins. "Why?" he wondered.

To answer his questions, Dad had several armadillos shipped to the Boston Lying-In, but the hospital did not have any facilities for keeping animals. He solved that problem—he thought—by building a small enclosure for the armadillos in the morgue's autopsy room. One morning at about 3 a.m., however, he got a call from the hospital cook, whose kitchen was next to the autopsy room. "There's a terrible smell in the hallway," the cook complained, "and the odor is coming from the morgue!"

Nonchalantly, Dad advised the cook to place a fan in the doorway of the autopsy room to keep the odor away, and then he went back to sleep. When he arrived at work later that morning, he discovered what had happened—the armadillos had somehow gotten loose, overturned a vat of formalin, and were running free in the hospital basement on feet that smelled like embalming fluid. When I heard the story, I imagined my father running after these funny-looking animals in the hospital kitchen while an irate cook chased *him* with a cleaver! Whatever actually happened, Dad's only summary of the incident was, "Fortunately, the armadillos weren't hard to catch."

Dad found that the animal world offered other opportunities for learning. He began making weekly trips to Yale's medical school, where Don Barron, a professor of physiology, had established a unique sheep research center. Dad worked with Barron to understand why anencephalic fetuses had excess amniotic fluid. They discovered that sheep fetuses regulated their water intake and urination with pituitary secretion. This new information came contrary to the teaching of the top neonatologist at the Boston Lying-In Hospital.

Dad developed considerable respect for Don Barron and began to learn a great deal about what animals could teach an astute researcher. He also learned whom Dr. Barron considered a hero. One morning—on Tuesday, April 19, 1955—Dad arrived at Barron's lab with donuts, as was his weekly custom. Dr. Barron told him solemnly, "There will be no experiment today. *He* died last night." The "he" was Albert Einstein, whom Dr. Barron clearly revered.

Like a detective who couldn't stop solving crimes, Dad investigated more and more questions that called for answers. He wondered what agent would cause freemartin syndrome—a condition in which cows give birth to male and female twins and the female twin is sterile. He then questioned why marmosets, monkeys native to South America that nearly always have fraternal twins, were *not* born sterile. Dad was puzzled since unborn marmosets share placental blood vessels, like cows with freemartin syndrome do.

To investigate, my father began visiting Chicago stockyards to obtain the fetuses of freemartin cows. Then he decided to acquire marmosets as well as tamarins, both small primates from South America. During a cocktail party at our house one evening, one of Dad's connections from the zoo world delivered Max and Moritz, a pair of cotton-top tamarins. Since Harvard and its associated hospitals had no place to house a colony of primates, Dad decided to convert the cellar of our house into several floor-to-ceiling habitats, with trees for the monkeys to climb and a one-way viewing glass in the door for observation. He also established a beetle colony to help feed the tamarins and marmosets.

Zoos at the time often had problems breeding these primates, but for some reason, Dad had no trouble. Thanks to prolific breeding and more purchases, the Benirschke "zoo" grew to as many as 35 monkeys! They required frequent attention and feeding, so someone—most often Mom—always had to be home. If an animal was sick when Dad was traveling, his first question to Mom when calling home was *not* "How are you and the kids?" but "How is the sick monkey?"

Growing up as a child of Kurt Benirschke was never dull. Who else had monkeys in their basement? The tamarins and marmosets are among my most vivid early memories, and they helped inspire my own passion for animals. I loved taking friends down to the basement and showing off the monkeys. They were very active, jumping from tree to tree, and were fascinating to watch. We often hand-fed them mealworms, which we were also breeding in our beetle colony. One day a neighbor friend, Johnny Tyler, and I were feeding the tamarins and marmosets when he challenged me to eat a mealworm. What could I do? My five-year-old honor was at stake. I swallowed the mealworm whole and maintained the respect of the kids in the neighborhood.

I considered the monkeys almost part of the family. They were a source of enjoyment for several years, right up to the time we moved to New Hampshire and Dad found them new homes in various zoos.

With all his responsibilities at work and home, my father might have considered his plate full. But his interests and curiosity were compelling him to look in other directions. The field of genetics was already 50 years old, but it wasn't until the mid-1950s that technology had advanced enough to make it possible to obtain accurate counts of both human and animal chromosomes. Dad naturally wanted to know more. Soon, he was adding genetics to his expanding knowledge.

As the 1950s came to a close, he had spent nearly a decade in the Boston area. It seemed that he was poised to set down roots at the Lying-In Hospital. But an unexpected phone call and a surprising decision would lead to new adventures for Dad and our family—away from Boston.

PART 3
HANOVER

Animal Tales

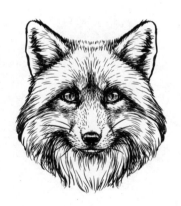

CHAPTER 7

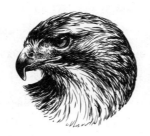

THE KINGDOM

Dartmouth College was founded in 1769 in Hanover, New Hampshire. Its 269 picturesque acres sit on the banks of the Connecticut River, which divides New Hampshire from Vermont, and its medical school is the fourth oldest in the country. One of its former faculty members, Supreme Court Justice Oliver Wendell Holmes Jr., introduced the stethoscope to the US medical curriculum.

Dad didn't know any of this in the summer of 1959 when he took a phone call from a friendly man named Marsh Tenney. As the new dean of Dartmouth's medical school, Tenney was charged with revitalizing the school. Would my father be interested, Tenney wondered, in becoming the pathology department chair?

Dad wasn't even sure where Hanover was when he first took the call from Tenney, and he certainly wasn't looking to move. As he later wrote, "We loved our house, the kids liked Wellesley, we earned enough to live, I loved my job—why leave?"

But Tenney was persuasive. After learning where Hanover was, Dad realized he had a short trip planned nearby in September, and he agreed to drop in and "take a look." He drove to Hanover on a lovely autumn day. On his way, he stopped to buy red apples from a roadside stand and enjoyed the lush countryside. In town, the sugar maples and hemlocks were displaying their fall colors, and Main Street was at its most charming. Hanover was making a good first impression.

The favorable impression continued during Dad's tour of the college and medical school. He enjoyed his conversations with Marsh Tenney and the other faculty and staff, and he returned home intrigued. A second visit, this time with Mom, also went well and led to an official offer for Dad to take over as chair of the pathology department.

It was a tough decision, not helped by the fact that some of Dad's colleagues thought he was crazy to even consider leaving. After all, they told him, Harvard was the most prestigious educational institution in the country. Why move to rural Dartmouth, a place that was only just starting to ramp up the quality of its medical school? They advised him that most of his colleagues would view it as a career step down. But my father had never been concerned about building the perfect résumé or, for that matter, what others thought about him or his plans. He simply wanted the best opportunities to learn and pass on his knowledge to others. The more he thought about it, the more he liked the idea of having the freedom to make his own mark in a town where everything seemed to revolve around the college.

After much soul-searching, Dad accepted the position, which would start in July 1960. At age 36, he would be the youngest chair in the history of the school's pathology department, and foreign-born to boot. On one of his follow-up visits to Hanover, he brought Mom, and she found a house that was perfect for our family—within walking distance of the school that we kids would attend.

Meanwhile, the pathology department at Dartmouth was also in the process of moving. Construction workers were just finishing a new medical school building. Dad's early days were filled with meeting new colleagues and learning the duties required of a department head. The transition was doubly intense because the previous pathology chair had died in a plane crash and other key faculty members had resigned. Dad was left to rebuild the department on his own. Making matters even more complicated, he had just two months to prepare a course on pathology for incoming students. This was especially daunting since he had never taught a course in his life. But, in his typical fashion, Dad figured it out.

He hired two new faculty members, one of them from Germany, and dove into studying the existing pathology curriculum, barely staying ahead of his students in the reading as he taught the course. Convinced from his early work at Harvard that the department needed an emphasis on reproductive pathology, he successfully applied for a National Institutes of Health grant with the help of Henry Heyl, a medical school associate who would become one of his closest friends at Dartmouth. Soon both the department and the students were flourishing. Dad was already beginning to leave his mark.

Our family was also enjoying New Hampshire. Hanover's 7,000 residents took full advantage of the outdoors and the wonderful opportunities that came with the change of seasons. The town averaged nearly 70 inches of snowfall each year, so snow was a major part of our lives. My parents found some skis and parkas for each of us at a fall swap meet, and we started learning how to ski on a small slope in front of our house. We graduated to steeper slopes and, thanks to a ski program taught after school by local parents, we grew to love the sport. Dad was the least proficient, as he simply didn't have the time to learn, but he was enthusiastic and took us skiing as often as he could.

Once during a family outing at the Dartmouth Skiway, Dad was trying to keep up with Steve and me and fell on a particularly steep section of the trail. He didn't know it at the time, but his car keys fell out of his pocket. It wasn't until the end of the day, when we were packing up and ready to drive home and he couldn't find his keys, that he realized what must have happened. By then, the lifts were closed and it was starting to get dark. Dad, Steve, and I grudgingly trudged back up the slope to look for the keys. Just as it was getting too dark to see, we miraculously found them at the site where he had fallen. We teased Dad about that for the rest of his life. (Even as I write this, I can't help but chuckle.)

The snow affected our lives in other ways. Our relatively flat roof had to be shoveled regularly, as did the driveway. We usually didn't mind, except when the big street snowplow clearing the main road drove by just after we had finished shoveling our long driveway. It invariably left a huge berm of snow and ice that blocked the end of the driveway and required us to go back out and clear it again.

During the spring and summer, my siblings and I could ride our bicycles or walk home from school. Most days we took a shortcut across the Dartmouth athletic fields where teams practiced soccer, football, or lacrosse. We often retrieved balls for the players and stayed to hang out and watch. If we were lucky, one of the players would play catch with us for a minute or two. They instantly became our favorite players, and we would watch when the games started and follow the progress of their college careers.

We didn't own a television growing up—my father didn't believe in "wasting time" on trivial entertainment—so we entertained ourselves by going outside. Both Steve and I got into whatever sport was in season: soccer in the fall, ski racing and ice hockey in the winter, and baseball and tennis in the spring and summer. Ingrid fell in love with figure skating. We were an active family that appreciated the sound and feel of being outdoors—the crunch of hard snow beneath our boots, the exhilaration of skiing and making the first tracks down the mountain, the experience of lacing up our skates and gliding across a frozen pond while passing a puck back and forth with a friend.

We loved our home in Hanover—but another piece of property would help us create memories that would shape us and open our eyes to the world around us.

CHAPTER 7: THE KINGDOM

∞

The poet John Greenleaf Whittier, a native of Massachusetts, once wrote: "New England is full of Romance. . . . We have mountains pillaring a sky as blue as that which bends over classic Olympus; streams as bright and beautiful as those of Greece and Italy; and forests richer and nobler than those which of old were haunted by Sylph and Dryad."

I don't know that Dad was thinking of the romance of New England's mountains, streams, and forests when he started looking at property-for-sale ads in backcountry newspapers during those first years in Hanover. His motivation was more about finding a place for our family to get away from it all. Many other families we knew took a vacation once or twice a year, but my parents didn't do vacations. Instead, we piled into our Buick station wagon and traveled with Dad to his conferences, speaking engagements, and business meetings.

One day, Dad found a piece of property while looking through the newspaper. The Kingdom, as he later named it, was an old homestead built in the 1800s. It included a small house and a couple of broken-down barns on 200 acres at the top of a long dirt road in the middle of Vermont, about 25 miles from our home. It was rundown and had no electricity or running water. But the land was gorgeous, with 100 acres of fields surrounded by another 100 acres of green woods and undisturbed wildlife. With little deliberation, Dad bought it for $4,000, a significant sum for us at the time. For a family like ours that enjoyed the outdoors, the Kingdom was a kind of paradise, a place that indeed captured the romance of New England. It was both "bright and beautiful" and "richer and nobler."

During our first weekends there, we developed a routine. We would leave Hanover and head toward the Kingdom late on a Friday afternoon. Along the way, we'd stop to watch a drive-in movie in one of the little towns we passed through, usually a western featuring John Wayne or a James Bond film with Sean Connery playing the role of 007. After the show, we would continue the short drive that ended on a dirt road leading up the hill to the house. Then we would make popcorn on the wood-burning stove and relax before crawling into bed. We spent the next two days exploring the fields and woods or fixing up our home away from home. It was a lot of work, and we all helped with throwing out old junk; tearing down one of the barns; repairing windows, doors, and floors; putting up new pine-paneled walls inside and clapboard outside; painting; and more.

For a boy not quite 10 years old, the Kingdom was a fascinating place that invited exploration. When I wasn't helping with repairs or camping in a tent in the yard, I was venturing into the fields and woods. I learned where the deer and foxes made their homes, found woodchuck dens, and discovered where the ruffed grouse liked to hang out. I loved sneaking up on the grouse to see how close I could get. Dad taught us how to shoot a rifle, and we hunted some woodchucks and had lots of target practice competitions.

My favorite activity, though, was discovering and watching the amazing birds on our property. I'd taken up birding back in Hanover, often going on walks with my friend Brookes Morin. We had competed over who could see and identify a bird first. I carried Roger Tory Peterson's classic book *A Field Guide to the Birds* everywhere I went. Before dinner each night, I'd read and learn everything I could about the characteristics of various birds and how to tell them apart, their range, and more. (To this day, I constantly scan the tops of trees or power line poles, looking for whatever hawk or falcon might be sitting on them.) At the Kingdom, I had a whole new area to explore and new birds to add to my growing "life list" of birds I'd seen in person.

Once the house was in better shape, Dad started driving up to the Kingdom for quiet weekends to work on his writing. He was still consumed by his many other responsibilities and interests, among them his continuing investigations of the placenta. It was becoming even more apparent to him that the placenta was a key organ that could reveal many insights about maternal and fetal health and disease.

Dad realized the need for a central resource where all of this new information could be found. He took advantage of the peace and quiet at the Kingdom to write the first volume of the *Pathology of the Human Placenta*. It was, he wrote, a "deliberate attempt to bring together the practical information which has been gathered about the pathology of this complex organ and to make it available to the practicing pathologist as well as clinician." His book became the authoritative text in the field, and the textbook is still used in medical schools everywhere. It became an ongoing project to describe new discoveries as they were made. Dad produced five more editions of the book over the next 45 years, giving doctors and researchers an invaluable resource for decades.

I went to the Kingdom with my father whenever he would let me. Making the long drive up the hill was always special since inevitably we would see something interesting. I'd say, "Dad, look at that!" after spotting a porcupine, or "Dad, stop, stop! See those deer over there?" We both watched for birds as well. I often corrected him when he saw one and guessed what it was, telling him, "No, Dad, that's not a red-tail, that's a Cooper's hawk." He knew so much about seemingly everything that I gained some extra satisfaction when I felt like more of an expert on something than he was. I knew my birds.

The road to the Kingdom wound through fields that were bordered by the Connecticut River on one side and deep woods on the other, perfect habitat for deer and foxes and all kinds of other interesting animals. Unfortunately, the wildlife was sometimes hit by passing cars. With Dad's lifelong work in medicine and pathology, he saw that as an invitation for more learning. Whenever we found dead wildlife, we would stop to examine it—a fox, porcupine, opossum, deer, weasel. But that was only the start of our education. Often, we would also wrap up the head of the animal and take it home. We then boiled the head in a big pot on our stove at home—much to my mother's dismay—until it became a white skull. Dad used the skulls to teach us about the anatomy of the wildlife, and then he put them in large, framed collections that filled bookshelves in his study. To her credit, Mom eventually got used to it all—though she would often shake her head in mock disgust every time we showed up with a new skull. The collection was later donated to the Natural History Museum in San Diego.

I read lots of westerns and had already developed a love of the outdoors through the pages of books, but it was on that farm and in those fields that my lifelong passion for nature and wildlife was cemented. Dad enjoyed hosting annual picnics there for the Dartmouth medical students he was teaching, and it was always a special treat to have birthday parties at the farm. I think it was fulfilling for him to see his children delight in being there. As he later wrote, "It was one of the happy times in our family's life." At the farm, my siblings and I learned "how to appreciate animals and the quiet and the beauty of nature." Dad felt that delight and appreciation too. He wrote, "We loved the evenings with deer coming out of the woods to graze, watching the foxes sneaking up on something, and to behold the absolute stillness of the Kingdom." The spirit of New England must have captured him, because he added, "At times, the place appeared romantic to us. While we had it, we loved it."

In later years, Dad embraced some of the sayings of Chief Seattle, a Suquamish and Duwamish Native American chief in the 1800s. One of the most famous quotes attributed to the chief was, "Humankind has not woven the web of life. We are but one thread within it. Whatever we do to the web, we do to ourselves. All things are bound together."

The idea that we are all bound together in this world—animals, plants, and humans—was already a growing part of Dad's philosophy when he purchased our little piece of paradise in Vermont. Our time there further solidified this way of looking at the world. This worldview would influence the rest of my father's days and yield far-reaching results.

CHAPTER 8

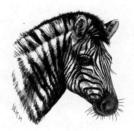

Counting Chromosomes

I n 1952, a Chinese American cell biologist named T. C. Hsu accidently washed a culture of cells with a hypotonic solution rather than the isotonic saline solution he intended to use. When Hsu looked at the cells, he found that the chromosomes were spread out so well on his microscope slide that they were easy to count. As so often happens in science, that one mistake led to a significant breakthrough. With Hsu's discovery, it became possible for the first time to obtain accurate counts of structures that contained genetic material. Scientists using Hsu's hypotonic technique reported that the number of chromosomes in humans was not 48, as had been believed for three decades, but 46! A new field of science, cytogenetics—the study of chromosomal structure, location, and function in cells—was born.

My father was fascinated and excited by this development when he read about it in one of the many journals he devoured every month. He wondered, "If we developed a better understanding of our genetic makeup, would that also tell us about disease and other abnormalities?" Surely cytogenetics could answer important questions and lead to improved health for humans.

His questions and musings didn't stop there. Most scientists viewed human and animal medical issues as separate and largely unrelated fields, but Dad's previous research on armadillos and marmosets had shown close parallels with human biology and function. If all things were "bound together," as Chief Seattle had suggested, then what might more research on the chromosomes of animals reveal to benefit all species? Dad resolved to find out.

Never shy about taking on a new challenge, Dad decided to address a question that had perplexed humanity for some 3,000 years. The mule—the product of a male donkey and a female horse—was the most common and oldest-known manmade hybrid animal. Combining the size of a horse with the strength, endurance, and patient disposition of a donkey, the mule had long served humans as an ideal choice for farm work and transporting cargo. To speed up the breeding process, people had tried for centuries to mate mules with one another, without success. The mystery as to why they wouldn't breed had never been solved. Why, except in the rarest of cases, were mules sterile?

Dad suspected that chromosomes might reveal the answer. Soon after arriving at Dartmouth, he was asked to give a talk on cytogenetics to a group of local pediatricians in Vermont. At the end of his lecture, he mentioned that he was interested in obtaining a blood sample of a mule and asked if anyone in the audience could help produce one. To his surprise, one of the pediatricians said he could. The next day, Dad and his colleague drove out to a farm owned by the pediatrician's friend. Once Dad agreed to pay the farmer $30 in case the mule accidentally died from the procedure, he was given permission to acquire a blood sample. It took a couple of tries—Dad wasn't used to inserting a needle through such thick skin—but he got the necessary blood sample, and the mule survived without a problem.

Back in his lab, Dad discovered that mules possessed 63 chromosomes. Once he confirmed that horses had 64 chromosomes and donkeys had just 62, he had his answer! The differences in structure and chromosome number prevented the chromosomes from pairing up properly, thus leaving the hybrid mule sterile. Dad published this important finding in the scientific journal *Fertility and Sterility*, and his passion for understanding chromosomes was born.

His next quest emerged from, of all places, a photo he discovered on the last page of a *Life* magazine. An issue published in October 1962 included an image of a donkey-like creature with black stripes on its white legs. Known as a "zebronkey," the hybrid animal had been born from a male zebra and a female donkey. Of course, Dad was intrigued. He later wrote, "Now that was an animal that was *really* worth learning more about. It presented a major challenge for our understanding of animal hybridization."

The zebronkey in the article was located at the Manila Zoo in the Philippines. Dad wondered how he could obtain a blood sample to learn more. He believed in the saying, "Luck favors the prepared mind," and it certainly applied in this case. He remembered that one of his former medical school residents from Boston lived in Manila, and, amazingly, her husband was on the Manila Zoo's board of trustees! Dad reached out to see if they could help acquire some blood, and they readily agreed.

It wasn't long before Dad received the precious sample in the mail. His interest was piqued when he looked at the zebronkey's chromosomes under a microscope. He knew that donkeys had 62 chromosomes, so he had expected the mother to contribute 31 to her zebronkey offspring—and she had. But Dad was astonished at the number of chromosomes contributed by the father, a zebra—only 16! This meant the zebra had just 32 chromosomes. At the time, every animal family he had studied showed the same or nearly the same chromosome count, regardless of the species. To find such a dramatic difference within equids—62 in the donkey and only 32 in the zebra—seemed unbelievable. Dad was equally surprised that the breeding had succeeded and that the hybrid had survived! He published a paper describing the startling results.

A few of his colleagues didn't seem to grasp the implications of this discovery and had some fun with his "eccentric" new interest, implying that a zebronkey wasn't a research subject worthy of a serious scientist. One of them was Dad's good friend T. C. Hsu, the biologist whose lab accident had led to an increase in the study of chromosomes. T. C. sent my father a cartoon he had drawn that depicted a daddy equine figure with vertical stripes, a mommy equine with horizontal stripes, and a baby equine with a checkerboard pattern. Dad took the good-natured ribbing in stride, but he wasn't going to let a few would-be comedians dampen his curiosity.

He was irritated, however, when he learned that his published paper contained an error. Authorities at the Manila Zoo had told him that the father of the hybrid was a Grevy's zebra, but knowledgeable readers wrote to say that the photo accompanying the paper clearly indicated that the father was actually a Hartmann's mountain zebra, a completely different species. He had no choice but to issue a correction—"not a happy event for any scientist"—the only one he ever had to submit during his career.

The error stirred Dad's curiosity even more, though. He wanted to examine the chromosome counts for all three known types of zebras: Grevy's, Hartmann's mountain, and plains zebras. (He learned over time that there are actually eight subspecies of zebras.) Once again, he faced a familiar challenge: since zebras made their homes in Africa, where could he obtain samples for study? The solution came through a fortunate mistake—one that would lead to a long and fruitful friendship.

∞

In the summer of 1963, our family piled into our Buick station wagon for another trip to one of Dad's speaking engagements, this time in Cincinnati. Steve, Ingrid, and I were especially excited because Dad planned to take us to Montreal immediately following his talk. He'd told us all kinds of wonderful things about the city and Canada, and we couldn't wait to get there.

As we were planning to leave the conference in Cincinnati to head up to Montreal, Dad realized he'd forgotten his passport. Because he'd only recently become a naturalized American citizen, he was worried about being allowed back into the United States if we went to Canada without his passport. Our trip to Montreal was suddenly off, but thankfully, the story did not end there.

That same evening, Dad bought a *Saturday Evening Post* magazine, which he hoped would help take our minds off our disappointment. In it, he found a fascinating article about the Catskill Game Farm in upstate New York. The game farm was the nation's first privately owned zoo. It featured close to 1,000 animals, including exotic wildlife, spread out over some 900 acres. The more my father read about the game farm, the more excited we all got. When he suggested we replace our Montreal trip with a visit to Catskill, we were practically jumping up and down with excitement.

Dad was happy to see his children smiling again, but he had another reason to be pleased about the unexpected schedule change—the game farm had zebras! Surely, he thought, this was a place where he could finally collect a few small zebra skin biopsies and learn more about different species of zebras.

We arrived at the Catskill Game Farm early the next morning and met Dr. Heinz Heck, the zoo director, and Roland Lindemann, the owner. Both were German, a good sign as far as Dad was concerned, and soon they were all speaking in German and getting along famously. While everyone got to know one another, Dad steered the conversation with Dr. Heck to the possibility of obtaining samples from the zebras. The answer was not what he'd hoped.

"No way," Dr. Heck said. "So many scientists have come. They want one piece of tissue or another, and it is never for the benefit of the animals. Nor do we ever hear of the outcome of their research after they leave. Sorry, you can't have any tissue. But you are welcome to visit the park."

Dad was disappointed, but he tried not to show it as we toured the game farm and enjoyed seeing the many different animals. The game farm gave the animals lots of room to roam and interact in natural ways. The arrangement also led to success with breeding.

We finished our day in the park and were headed for the exit when Dr. Heck caught up to us. "Herr Benirschke," he said to Dad, "I have been thinking about your request. Perhaps there is something that can be done, providing you would be willing to help me with a problem that I wish to have explored." It seemed that the Catskill director wanted to identify the genetic ancestry of American camelids, a family of animals that includes camels, llamas, and alpacas. Naturally Dad was willing to help. It was the beginning of a long-term friendship with the Catskill Game Farm that benefited everyone involved.

Dad got his zebra samples and determined that the Grevy's zebra had 46 chromosomes, the plains zebra had 44 chromosomes, and the Hartmann's mountain zebra had just 32. Armed with this new understanding, he was not content to stop with studying zebras. Now that he had a source for collecting samples, he was eager to utilize it. Fortunately, he had a couple of affordable and enthusiastic assistants ready to join him anytime he wanted to visit—Steve and me. Over the next several years, we made at least three trips annually to the Catskill Game Farm. Steve and I both enjoyed going and were always enthralled with watching the colorful peacocks wander the grounds, strutting their stuff. We loved searching for long tail feathers on the ground to bring home to Mom and Ingrid. Dad got on well with Dr. Heck, Roland Lindemann, and the staff, not just because they could speak German together but because they shared a common passion for helping and learning more about wildlife.

The process of obtaining samples was exciting for all of us. Even though the Catskill animals got a lot of exercise, many of the ungulates didn't get enough to properly wear down their hooves. About once a year, a zoo veterinarian needed to tranquilize the animals to give the staff a chance to trim their hooves or nails and do whatever else might be needed to keep the animals healthy. At those moments, Dad, Steve, and I often hustled to get a small blood sample and to clip a tiny piece of skin off an animal's ear or other accessible body part to "grow" later in the lab.

The technique of tranquilizing animals was relatively new and more of an art than a science at the time; veterinarians were often uncertain about the exact drug dosages to use. We never knew when a previously sedated, sleeping rhinoceros might suddenly open its eyes and not take kindly to us snipping off a small piece of its skin for a scientific sample. As a result, we learned to be quick and light on our feet.

Our efforts at the Catskill Game Farm became an important first step to cataloging the genetic makeup of many rare and endangered animals. One of Dad's most important discoveries from his involvement with the game farm included the Przewalski's horse, also known as the Mongolian wild horse. This beautiful and powerful animal, named after Russian geographer and explorer Nikolai Przewalski, was the world's oldest and last truly wild horse, but sadly it was on the verge of extinction in its native habitat. The prevailing belief was that the Przewalski's horse was an ancestor to domestic horses, but Dad discovered that this rare horse had 66 chromosomes, rather than 64 chromosomes like domestic horses had. This was strong evidence that the Przewalski's horse was actually a separate species. My father caused a big stir in the scientific community when he published his findings in *Science* in 1965. It led him to attend an international conference on the Przewalski's horse in East Berlin. Years later, DNA sequencing confirmed that the Przewalski's horse did indeed have its own distinct lineage.

Once Dad got started on establishing the importance of the karyotype—the number and appearance of chromosomes of an organism or species of animal—he couldn't stop. Our regular visits to the Catskill Game Farm continued, and more samples were taken from all kinds of wildlife. We also continued making sudden car stops at the sight of dead wildlife on the road so that Dad could get a skin sample for study. In addition, he began encouraging his colleagues to send him samples from rare animals in far-off places that he couldn't get to on his own. They were happy to oblige.

As a result of this important work, Dad and T. C. Hsu coauthored a book, *An Atlas of Mammalian Chromosomes*, published in 1967. The first volume of what would become an annual publication, it listed 50 species and included common and scientific names, taxonomic position, chromosome number, descriptions of autosomes and sex chromosomes, and the technique used for examining specimens. Dad and Dr. Hsu committed to publishing the chromosomes of 50 new species every year. The atlas became an invaluable resource for cytogeneticists everywhere, and it helped launch Dad's quest to learn more about endangered wildlife.

CHAPTER 9

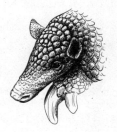

A Grand Expedition

A jeep transporting a rifle and machete, sausage, cans of gasoline, and four men bounced down a clay road in the wilderness. On each side of the road, *jacarés* (crocodiles) patrolled deep ditches filled with water left over from recent heavy rains. Countless herons, storks, caracaras (large falcons), and other birds perched in the abundant trees or flew overhead in the skies. The jeep's passengers—my dad, fellow pathologist Ralph Richart, a German lawyer they'd befriended, and a driver-guide—were traveling on the Ruta Transchaco, the "highway" leading into the vast Gran Chaco region of western Paraguay in South America. The four men were entering a sparsely populated and remote area known for its ecological diversity that featured both dense, dry forests and dusty, arid terrain. The Chaco was also known for being dangerous. Jaguars, venomous snakes, and drug runners ranged across the land, while flesh-eating piranhas searched for prey in the rivers.

Dad was a long way from his office and lab at Dartmouth. While he looked like a classic scientist in the lab with his white coat and microscope, Kurt Benirschke was hardly the stereotypical scientist. If he wasn't part Indiana Jones, then perhaps he was cut from the same mold as Teddy Roosevelt, another confident leader who combined his passions for science, nature, and adventure.

The goal of this trip, which began in May 1965, was to identify areas where different species of armadillos overlapped on the continent. It turned into a grand expedition that ignited Dad's lifelong love affair with South America and Paraguay in particular. By the time he and Ralph began their journey into the Chaco, they had already explored parts of Brazil. Now, riding in the hot jeep, Dad intently scanned the forest. He observed different types of cacti and many floss silk trees, known as *palo borracho*, which were covered with thorns and had swollen trunks that gave them the appearance of giant bottles. Finally, he spotted what he was looking for: a tree with a spreading canopy of finely pointed twigs and glistening, pointed, myrtle-like leaves—a quebracho tree! This was the same species of tree that produced the logs he'd once seen being unloaded at the docks in his native Glückstadt, Germany. The trees had originated right here! The stamps from Paraguay that my father eagerly collected as a boy had often led him to dream about this faraway place. Now, he was experiencing it for himself. Dad almost couldn't believe his good fortune, and he took a moment to reflect on how his life had come full circle. How lucky was he that he actually got to do the things he had so often wondered about?

The travelers motored deeper into the bush, successfully passing through checkpoints manned by young Paraguayan soldiers with rifles. In the late afternoon, they reached what must have looked like a mirage: a town in the middle of nowhere, complete with a museum, library, radio station, and hospital, along with streetlights and homes lined with white picket fences. The town, called Filadelfia, was a community of more than 10,000 Mennonites. Dad had read about the Mennonites' history. Their ancestors were Russian Mennonites who had been displaced during the Russian Revolution in 1917. They had first moved to Germany, then to Paraguay in 1930. The government had allowed them to settle deep in the Chaco where nobody else wanted to live, free from control but also from assistance. Appreciative of the opportunity and undaunted by the harshness of the land, the industrious Mennonites built the town of Filadelfia, carved out of the dense and unforgiving Chaco. There, they developed their own sources for power, water, and food and became totally self-sufficient. *And* they spoke German! Dad was delighted to learn that he could communicate with them directly—not just in German, but in *Plattdeutsch*, the dialect he had spoken while growing up in Glückstadt.

Over the next two days, the men toured the town of Filadelfia and explored the surrounding area, looking for indigenous wildlife. They caught a three-banded armadillo as part of their agreement with the Paraguayan government, encountered three large, venomous snakes, and visited a local doctor whose wife played Bach sonatas on a spinet.

Dad, his friends, and the armadillo departed Filadelfia early the next morning for the long drive on the dusty Ruta Transchaco back to Asunción, the nation's capital. They thought their adventures on this trip were over until one of the jeep's tires suddenly went flat and the gas tank was empty. Fortunately, the vehicle had just enough air and gasoline to limp into a *fortin* (military outpost). There, Dad and Ralph negotiated repairs on the tire by showing the post commander how to operate a Polaroid camera and gave the man a few pictures of himself. The group's driver, meanwhile, persuaded some of his former army buddies who were stationed at the post to loan him some gas for the next leg of their journey. With everything taken care of and thanks expressed all around, Dad and Ralph said goodbye to their lawyer friend and continued to Asunción, arriving early that evening.

When they checked into the Hotel Paraguay, Dad and Ralph couldn't wait to enjoy a well-earned dinner in the open-air restaurant that featured a "magnificent" harp performance. They went to their room, put the armadillo in the bathtub, and shut the door to the bathroom. Then they eagerly went back downstairs. Dad and Ralph enjoyed their food, sipped beer, and relived some of the trip's amazing experiences—totally unaware that several of the hotel's other guests weren't having such a relaxing evening. Apparently, the armadillo had gotten out of the bathtub, and from the outside hallway, a dog belonging to one of the guests had heard it scratching at the bathroom door. The excited dog was barking and trying to claw its way into the room. On their return from dinner, my dad and his friend were met with perturbed and excited guests and staff. It took some time to calm everyone down and explain that an armadillo was inside their room. They explained that they were studying the armadillo in the name of science and the animal would later be released back into its native habitat.

One of my father's few regrets in life was that he didn't become more familiar with Spanish, Portuguese, and other languages of South America. It would have helped him on this and subsequent trips—and saved him some embarrassment. On the day after the armadillo incident, in a meeting with Paraguay's minister of the interior, Dad proudly explained that during their visit, he and his colleague had been looking for "*tatu*." He was using the Spanish word for armadillo, but he didn't know that in Guarani, the local dialect, *tatu* meant "vulva." Some uncomfortable confusion ensued, but once Dad's words were cleared up, the amused official ceremoniously presented him with a Spanish-Guarani dictionary, hoping it might help in the future.

Dad and Ralph's next destination was nearly 800 miles south: Buenos Aires, the capital of Argentina. The plan was to take a passenger boat down the Paraná River, but the authorities refused to let the men board when they arrived at the harbor on the morning of their departure. Apparently, when they had crossed into Paraguay a few days before, no one from the immigration office had been at the border to stamp their passports. Dad and Ralph had simply walked across the border and not given it another thought. Now, the harbor authorities were saying that without a stamped passport, they needed a special permit to board.

The situation turned into quite a scene, and, they learned afterward, some of the passengers who were already on the boat began to make bets as to whether Dad and Ralph would be allowed passage. Despite a lot of arguing and negotiating, the American pathologists were told they were not allowed to board.

Fortunately, a local pathologist who had come to see the Americans off on their journey suggested that they quickly drive to the other side of town. There, they could hire someone to row them across the river to where the boat would make its first stop—back in Argentina. With no time to lose, Dad and Ralph raced through Asunción and found a willing ferryman. The small boat sprang a leak halfway across the river, but it remained seaworthy long enough to deliver the men to their destination, albeit a little wet from the experience.

When they landed, the border police greeted them again and asked why they were there. The Argentine authorities were concerned that they lacked the proper stamp on their passports, but when the Americans explained what they were doing, the border officials were so impressed by their work that they happily carried Dad's and Ralph's luggage to the boat dock. They arrived just in time to get in line and catch the boat that was already rounding the bend of the river. This time they had no problems boarding. Although several of the passengers lost money on their bets, Dad and Ralph were welcomed onboard with smiles and laughs. As my father later wrote in his typically optimistic style, "Luck was really with us today, but then I didn't expect otherwise."

As the boat traveled down the Paraná River on its way to Buenos Aires, Dad and Ralph made a brief stop in the city of Corrientes, where Dad had been invited to give a speech at the university. The Americans visited the city and the grounds where Teddy Roosevelt had once fished for golden dorado many years before. Then they traveled to Buenos Aires and embarked on a 300-mile drive to a remote cattle ranch.

On the morning after they arrived at the ranch, Dad and Ralph found themselves mounted on horses with nothing but sheepskin saddles as they joined their hosts for a daylong ride through the Pampas—vast, grassy plains that extend from the Atlantic Ocean to the Andes Mountains. At one point during the ride, Dad disappeared from sight and didn't respond to loud calls from the party. Ralph and the others, knowing that my father was a novice rider, assumed he must have fallen off his horse and thought he might be hurt somewhere back on the trail. When they turned around to find him, they saw Dad suddenly emerge from the tall grass, holding a squirming animal by its tail. He had spotted a hairy armadillo (*Chaetophractus villosus*), usually a nocturnal animal sought locally for its hide, and had decided to jump off his horse and give chase. Ever prepared, he quickly took some blood and tissue samples from the armadillo, then released the startled animal. His comrades were impressed and more than a little relieved that he wasn't hurt.

The next adventure on the travelers' agenda was a planned boat voyage up the Amazon River, another lifelong dream for Dad. But since he'd been gone for over a month, he decided to first call home and check in. Later, he would wish he'd never made the call. When he connected with Mom, she reluctantly told him that Dartmouth's president wanted him to return home immediately to vote on a crisis that was happening at the medical school. Never one to shirk his responsibilities, Dad had to give Ralph the bad news that their great South American expedition was over, and they both headed home. Regrettably, other than from an airplane, Dad never did get another chance to see the Amazon River. To make matters worse, the "crisis" was resolved even before he made it home to vote.

Nonetheless, he'd thoroughly enjoyed his initial foray into the continent of South America, and he was enthralled by the rich diversity of its people, wildlife, and ecosystems. To my dad, the trip and the many opportunities it had presented also underscored the value of his carpe diem philosophy. As he later wrote to his children, "Seemingly small events shape the future and lead to great things—what is important is to take the first step and enjoy the moment. . . . Seize the day!"

CHAPTER 9: A GRAND EXPEDITION

Since Dad hadn't fully accomplished the scientific goal of his journey to South America on that first trip—to identify the regions where seven- and nine-banded armadillos both lived—he returned the next year and fulfilled his mission. Those two trips to South America made a huge impression on Dad, and he would return many times over the next few decades. Years later, he wrote that those trips were among his favorite memories—that he could "still smell the forest and feel the heat."

He certainly enjoyed the unpredictable adventure. But there was more to it than that. Those trips, along with his many other travels, influenced his expanding vision of the world. My father was growing increasingly aware of the many connections between humans and the animal world. This shaped his thinking and changed the direction of his life.

CHAPTER 10

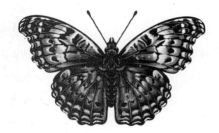

MOTHS AND ARMADILLOS

The thorny forests of South America may not have been a place to take young children, but Dad found other ways to share his love of traveling and investigating the animal world with his family. One was creating an extensive butterfly collection together. Everywhere we went, we kept a butterfly net in the car, and whenever we passed an open field or just needed a break from a long drive, we got permission to jump out and spend some time chasing butterflies. Dad also brought a net with him when he went on his travels to South America, bringing home some interesting butterflies in paper envelopes. It was my job to moisten their bodies so that when we spread their wings open to pin them on the "spreading board," the wings wouldn't break. We then mounted the butterflies in picture frames that showed off their brilliant colors. Over the years, we must have made at least 50 of those beautiful frames, exhibiting hundreds of butterflies from across the nation and around the world.

Exotic moths were also high on our list of fascinating winged insects to catch and display. One summer night when I was about eight years old, during a family trip to one of Dad's speaking engagements, we stopped at a two-story motel in Cleveland. As we got out of the car, I looked up and noticed a large moth sitting by a light on the outside wall near a second-floor room with a balcony.

I poked Steve and pointed excitedly. "See that moth?" I said. "It's huge. I wonder what it is."

This moth *was* a big one, over three inches long, with bright yellow wings, large antennae, and a large black spot on each of its hind wings. "Dad!" Steve called out. "You've got to see this!"

Dad stopped to look. "Beautiful," he said. "I think that's an Io moth. Do we have that in our collection?"

"No!" Steve and I answered in unison. "Dad," I added, "we gotta get this one! Do you think they'll let us into that upstairs room to try to catch it?"

When we all walked in, we saw a middle-aged man sitting behind the motel registration desk. "We'd like two rooms for the night, please," Dad said politely to the man, who appeared half asleep. "But I also have another request. Would you mind letting us into a room on the second floor so we can catch a moth that's right outside on the balcony?"

The motel clerk blinked, his bored expression turning into an incredulous frown. "What?" he said. "What are you talking about?"

"We collect butterflies and moths," Dad tried to explain, "and one of the kids saw a moth up there that we don't have in our collection."

"It's an Io moth," Steve said in his most helpful voice. "It's bright yellow and really big!"

The clerk blinked again. It appeared he was trying to decide if we were actually serious. "We may have a guest up there," he said a little reluctantly. "Where did you say it was?"

"They won't care!" I piped up. "I'm sure if we just knock on the door, they'll let us in."

After a bit more encouragement, the clerk figured out which room we were talking about and checked his registry. "Well, it actually looks like that room is empty," he said with a wry smile. "Why not? This is something I've got to see."

Steve and I went back to the car to grab a butterfly net and a jar we would need for the captured moth if we were successful. Finally, Dad, armed with the net, headed up the stairs to the second floor, followed by us three kids, with the now-curious clerk bringing up the rear. (Mom hung back, rolling her eyes about our latest "adventure.") When we got to the room, the clerk unlocked the door, and we all quietly slipped in. We passed through the room and tiptoed onto the balcony—the moth was still there. We almost couldn't believe our luck! We'd been searching for an Io moth for a long time and here it was, in the most unlikely of places. It took only a moment for Dad to sweep the net, capture the moth, and put it in the jar.

We all huddled around the colorful insect inside the jar. By now, the clerk seemed almost as excited as we were. "That's a big one, all right," he said. After we thanked him profusely and said goodnight, he walked away, still shaking his head, but now with a grin on his face. If nothing else, we'd certainly livened up his quiet summer evening.

As entertaining as the Io moth incident was, it did not come close in Benirschke family lore to the great Texas armadillo hunt. Our family, along with a Dartmouth medical student named John, took another "vacation" to Texas A&M University so Dad could check out what was supposedly a pregnant male armadillo. He ran some tests and determined the armadillo was not pregnant after all—no surprise. The next day, we drove to a ranch owned by a friend of Dad's near Huntsville, arriving in the late afternoon. Since nine-banded armadillos were plentiful in Texas, our goal was to catch a few that Dad could take back to Hanover to study and breed.

Dad's friend and his wife welcomed us into their home and offered us a Texas barbecue meal. Once it got dark, it was time to "hunt." Ingrid, who was about seven at the time, decided to stay and watch television, which was a rare treat for a Benirschke. The rest of us—Dad, Mom, Steve, me, John the medical student, and Dad's friend—made the trek to a neighbor's ranch armed with flashlights, a shovel, and some pillowcases that would hold the armadillos until they could be put in kennels for the trip home.

When we arrived, a weather-beaten gentleman wearing a cowboy shirt and jeans answered our knock on the door. "Hi, Joe," Dad's friend said to the rancher. "This here is Kurt, the doctor/scientist I was telling you about, and his wife, Marion, and their kids. They've come all the way down from New Hampshire and would like to go out into your pasture and catch some armadillos, if that's still all right with you."

Joe grunted. "Heck, yes," he said in a thick Texas drawl. "Those armadillos are always digging their holes on my land. I'm just waiting for one of my horses or cows to step into one and break a leg. You go ahead and take as many armadillos as you can catch. I just want to get rid of 'em. Just curious—what do you want those critters for, anyway?"

Dad began to explain his research, stating how armadillos had a single egg that always split into four identical embryos and produced identical quadruplets, something very rare in the animal world. After a few sentences, Joe raised his hand.

"Never mind, doctor, that's over my head," he said. "But you can go get as many as you want. I'll even loan you my dogs to help you flush 'em out and chase 'em into their burrows. Then it should be easy to dig 'em out."

Five minutes later, we all headed out into a huge field. Dad carried the shovel, Steve and John had the flashlights, Mom and I carried the pillowcases and rope, and Dad's friend held the leashes of three dogs that were sniffing the air and straining to run. The night was dark, but the stars were so bright that I could clearly make out the constellations. I was excited and a little nervous. Adult nine-banded armadillos are only about two to three feet long from head to tail and weigh about 12 pounds, but they have long, sharp claws on the middle toes of their forefeet. I knew they were powerful diggers, and none of us wanted them to use those claws on us!

The flashlights showed plenty of burrows in the ground, so we knew we were in the right place. A few moments later, Dad's friend released the dogs, which shot into the night like rockets, sniffing and barking as they ran. Suddenly, in the faint glow of our flashlight beams, we saw them come together to chase a dark creature scurrying across the field with surprising speed—an armadillo!

Dad quickly started to chase after the armadillo, his long legs churning as fast as they could go. He was running with his arms extended toward the ground—in the darkness he looked like a fast-moving zombie—when the wily armadillo dashed into a burrow and disappeared.

Dad stopped, bending over to catch his breath while the dogs barked, and started digging into the burrow. Just then, he spotted another armadillo and shouted: "There! Shine the light over there!" Soon he was running after another critter. Not to be outdone this time, he jumped and grabbed it by the tail just as the animal dove for its burrow. Dad fell to the ground but was still able to hold on. The armadillo's body was partially in its hole, but it was digging and squirming as hard as it could, trying to get away. The dogs, barking and jumping, gathered around Dad and the armadillo and watched as an unusual version of tug-of-war ensued, with my father pulling on the tail with both hands and the armadillo trying to escape into its hole.

"Tickle its belly!" Dad's friend instructed. "It will cause him to release his grip and he won't be able to dig anymore!"

Dad did as he was told, but the armadillo, apparently sensing its opportunity, lunged forward and escaped my dad's grip. With a grunt, the armadillo disappeared beneath the earth. Dad, who was again breathing hard, straightened and kicked the ground.

Armadillos 2, Benirschkes 0.

A minute later, however, Dad was in hot pursuit of another fast, zigzagging armadillo, with the dogs, Steve, and me chasing after them. "Jump on it like it's a football fumble!" shouted our host.

"If only Kurt knew what a football was," Mom chuckled from the darkness.

Dad ignored both of them, intent on redeeming himself. Suddenly he dove to the ground again. A moment later, Steve's flashlight showed Dad triumphantly holding a squirming armadillo by the tail, the grin on his face a mile wide.

"That's one!" he said as Steve and I cheered and the dogs barked even louder. "Here, Rolfie, bring one of those pillowcases." I ran over and opened up a pillowcase, holding it as far away from my body as possible, while he dropped in the wriggling mammal. We had finally bagged our first armadillo!

The hunt continued into the night. If someone happened to be driving by the ranch that evening, they would have observed quite a spectacle—men and boys and dogs running crazily around the field in wild, zigzag patterns, flashlight beams bouncing about and occasionally illuminating dark little forms scurrying here and there, accompanied by excited shouts and barks. It must have looked like a scene from a comedy or horror movie—or both. I can only imagine what the rancher was thinking as he watched us.

By the time the great hunt was over, we'd successfully captured six armadillos in pillowcases and quickly transferred them to kennels so we could ship them back to New Hampshire. Everyone was exhausted but happy with the outcome of the evening.

Everyone except perhaps Mom, who, as we drove away, said something quietly about needing to buy some new pillowcases.

CHAPTER 11

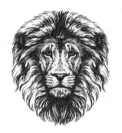

Ahead of His Time

My father, Kurt Benirschke, was increasing his focus on both human and animal chromosomes and other genetic projects. He continued to be curious about the problems and diseases connected to reproduction, particularly as they related to the birth of twins, and his studies of the placenta were advancing. Every new discovery or insight was exciting to him, but expanding his personal knowledge base was never enough. It remained vitally important to Dad that his discoveries—and the discoveries of others—were published so the entire world would benefit from new advances in medicine. He was already working on what would become part of his life's work: *Pathology of the Human Placenta* and *An Atlas of Mammalian Chromosomes*. Even so, he continued to look for other ways to get the word out.

It was in 1965, during discussions at a meeting of the National Academy of Sciences' Committee on Pathology, that Dad had the idea to create a series of international conferences that would explore his diverse-yet-related interests.

Dartmouth would host the first weeklong conference in 1966, focused on "Comparative Reproductive Failure." He invited accomplished doctors and researchers from both human medical and veterinary realms, including Arthur Hertig, chair of Harvard Medical School's pathology department; E. S. E. Hafez, professor at Washington State University's reproduction laboratory; M. C. Chang, reproductive biologist at the Worcester Foundation for Experimental Biology; and John King, veterinary officer and head of the capture unit of the game department in Nairobi, Kenya.

In a publication about the first conference, Dad later wrote, "It was felt that investigators in medicine and the veterinary fields would profit greatly from a closer liaison. All too frequently, we work relatively isolated in our respective fields and, with the burgeoning information filling our journals, we have not enough time and leisure to stand back and attempt a comparative look at the subject of study. Often, we are not familiar with the techniques other disciplines use, and which we could well employ to great advantage."

The conference was a success, attracting considerable interest from leaders in a variety of fields. The scientific publishing company Springer-Verlag created a book nearly 500 pages long from the conference. The book featured 28 papers and other presentations, including "Genetic and Biochemical Aspects of Reproductive Failure," "Comparative Aspects of Steroid Hormones in Reproduction," and my dad's own contribution, "Sterility and Fertility of Interspecific Mammalian Hybrids." Plans were soon underway for a second conference, this time on the West Coast.

The next summer, our family prepared for another Benirschke-style "vacation" by loading our station wagon to the brim with suitcases, tents, sleeping bags, butterfly nets, and more to begin a monthlong trip that would take us more than 6,000 miles round trip from our home in New Hampshire. Our destination was Washington State University in Pullman, the location for the second international conference, where Dad would speak again. Our drive there took us through Canada and included stops in Montreal, Toronto, and Edmonton, along with many other sites along the Trans-Canada Highway. On the trip back, we toured the northern United States and passed through Montana, Yellowstone National Park, and, of course, the Catskill Game Farm before finally returning home. It was a trip full of memories we kids would never forget.

The international conference was held again in 1968, this time at Dartmouth, where the subject was "Comparative Mammalian Cytogenetics," a topic Dad had grown especially interested in. Once again, he assembled an impressive array of speakers and guests, including his friend T. C. Hsu and geneticist and evolutionary biologist Susumu Ohno from the City of Hope Medical Center in Duarte, California. Some of the papers presented and later published at this third conference included "Mechanisms of Chromosome Speciation in Mammalian Speciation," "Induced Chromosomal Aberrations with Special Reference to Man," and "Consideration of Sex Chromosome Abnormalities in Man." Dad also presented his paper, coauthored with R. J. Low and V. H. Ferm, titled "Cytogenetic Studies of Some Armadillos," which included information he learned from his research on the armadillos we had caught during our eventful trip to Texas.

A subsequent book featured other presentations from the conference. In the foreword, Dad included a quote from British physician and naturalist R. B. Seymour Sewell that prodded his colleagues to think about the meaning of what they were doing: "It has been said that scientists in this search for truth are nowadays too much concerned with the accumulation of facts and make too little use of their imagination in their attempts to explain such facts as they have accumulated." Like Sewell, my father was always thinking ahead, always looking for the meaning and benefit of each new revelation.

It was around this time that a stunning nature documentary stirred his imagination. *The Last Paradises*, released in Germany in 1967, was the product of seven years of filmmaking by director and producer Eugen Schuhmacher and cinematographer Helmuth Barth. The filmmakers had traveled to 60 countries and territories around the world to film rare and never-before-seen footage of endangered wildlife in their native habitats. The Javan rhinoceros and the Hamilton's frog were both portrayed on film for the first time. The film also depicted shoebill storks, Kodiak bears, whooping cranes, Asiatic lions, Komodo dragons, and birds-of-paradise, along with many other spectacular animals.

The documentary moved my dad. He later wrote that it made a lasting impression and was "clearly the most beautiful film I had ever seen." It wasn't just the amazing cinematography that inspired him. The movie revealed some of the most beautiful wildlife on the planet and highlighted how close the world was to losing these remarkable animals. To a scientist who had already learned to appreciate the value and diversity of all wildlife, the film was virtually a call to arms.

Dad got in touch with the German embassy and received approval to borrow the film so he could show it during the 1968 international conference at Dartmouth. He then rented Hanover's local movie house, the Nugget Theater on Main Street, and Steve, Ingrid, and I stood at the entrance of the old brick building to collect donations from conference-goers and other patrons to help cover costs. The movie was powerful, but in the late 1960s, few people were talking about endangered wildlife or loss of habitats, let alone taking steps to do anything about it. Dad was ahead of his time . . . again.

After seeing *The Last Paradises*, he now felt an urgent need to communicate his growing concern over threats to wildlife and habitats around the world. It didn't take long before he found a way to take action.

Dad had heard about a new "miracle drug" being used by veterinarians in Africa to sedate animals that required wound treatment, dental care, vaccinations, and other important procedures. The drug was a significant breakthrough, as it was difficult for veterinarians to estimate just the right dosage for the muscle relaxants used up to this time. Too small a dose and the animal might jump to its feet prematurely, potentially threatening the caregivers (a danger Steve and I were quite familiar with, thanks to our time at the Catskill Game Farm); too large a dose and the animal might develop breathing difficulties, potentially endangering its life. The new drug, known as M99, was a morphine analogue that acted to immobilize an animal without the risk of breathing problems. It could also be combined with a recovery agent that revived the "patient" with a shot. The new drug hadn't yet been approved for use in the United States, but evidence of its success was beginning to spread.

Dad invited John King, a veterinarian and game department official from Kenya, to the second Dartmouth conference. He urged King to discreetly bring a supply of M99 so he could observe this new agent for himself. Following the conference, he and King made a trip to the Catskill Game Farm, where they planned to test the drug. After putting several precautions in place, Roland Lindemann allowed the two men to inject a zebra, an onager, and a llama that needed routine procedures. They used the M99, then "woke up" each animal with the recovery agent. In all three cases, the drugs performed beautifully, with no ill effects on the animals. Dad and the game farm staff were delighted; they realized this was an important new development that would benefit animals and their caregivers across the country and around the world.

It was the following year that my father would use our family as "mules" to smuggle M99 and an immobilization pistol across Checkpoint Charlie, behind the Iron Curtain, and into East Berlin, where the items would finally reach the staff at Tierpark Berlin. Dad had no patience for bureaucracy. He'd personally seen the effects of M99 and knew it would be approved eventually for worldwide use. Why wait? In his mind, the benefits clearly outweighed the risks.

Dad had visited the Antwerp Zoo in Belgium in the early 1960s, impressing the staff there by performing a biopsy on a Przewalski's horse hybrid that had produced sperm (and presumably could reproduce). The zoo director then invited him to speak at the 125th anniversary of the zoo in 1968. The topic was the importance of doing research in zoos.

At the anniversary ceremonies, Dad's presentation went well. He was especially excited about one listener in the room: Charles R. Schroeder, DVM, better known to friends and colleagues as "Charlie." Charlie Schroeder was known throughout the animal world as the visionary director of the highly regarded San Diego Zoo. Like Dad, Charlie was ahead of his time on the topics of conservation of endangered wildlife and habitat preservation. Charlie had spoken for years on the need to take action, and he had some ideas about what needed to be done closer to home in San Diego.

When Dad and Charlie met at the Antwerp Zoo, they hit it off. They spent a lot of time touring the zoo there and discussing what they might do to help preserve endangered species. Soon after, Dad scheduled a trip to San Diego to discuss a potential grant with Scripps Research and to meet again with Charlie at the Zoo. Charlie wondered if Dad would be willing to talk about M99 and show the film he had taken at the Catskill Game Farm to the veterinarians at the San Diego Zoo. His answer, of course, was an enthusiastic yes!

"I challenged the vets to see the drug as the anesthetic of choice for the future sedating of animals," Dad shared later. "They didn't take me very seriously at first, even laughing at it, but Charlie did. He supported my efforts to import and legalize the drug. M99 has since been modified, and new drugs have come along, but it was the first drug to offer this life-saving option to vets and animal care staff everywhere."

Dad's life had been an interesting adventure, taking him from war medic to pathologist, from medical school instructor to expert on the placenta and genetics. Now, it was increasingly leading him into the realms of wildlife, conservation, and zoos.

PART 4
SAN DIEGO

ONE MEDICINE

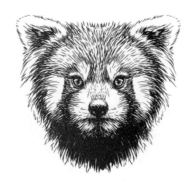

CHAPTER 12

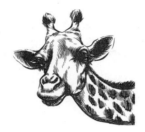

CALIFORNIA OR BUST

It was Christmas Eve 1969, and a gentle snowfall was silently adding to the four feet of white that already blanketed our yard and home in Hanover. Inside the house, our family had just enjoyed the wonderful goose dinner Mom had cooked. One of Dad's favorite meals, it reminded him of his home in Glückstadt and was always followed with a plum pudding dessert that was dressed in warm brandy and set alight. Dinner was always slow and leisurely on Christmas Eve—an annoying tradition for Steve, Ingrid, and I, who tried to hurry our parents along so we could get to the wrapped presents under the Christmas tree. That evening, we all helped Mom clear the dining room table after the meal, and the kids dried the dishes as she washed.

Christmas was my favorite holiday for many reasons, but one of the big ones was that the vacation gave me a lot of time to play ice hockey. I was 14 years old and a freshman in high school. Our bantam hockey team from little Hanover had just knocked off several bigger and more experienced teams and was about to win the New Hampshire state championship. I wanted to finish drying the dishes because I hoped one of the presents under the tree was a new pair of hockey skates. Steve was also working quickly. He nudged me and asked, "Can't we get Mom and Dad to hurry up? They're even slower than usual this year! I wonder what's up." I shrugged. I had no idea.

As we were finishing with the dishes, Dad walked into the kitchen and whispered something into Ingrid's ear. They both slipped out of the room. Steve and I noticed but didn't think much about it. We were too focused on getting the dishes done as quickly as possible so we could head into the living room. A few minutes later, Dad returned and loudly cleared his throat.

"I have something to tell the family," he said rather dramatically.

Just then, Ingrid walked in behind him holding up a large poster. In words she had just neatly written, it read, "California or Bust!" Both she and Dad had strange smiles on their faces as they watched our reactions.

"What is this?" Steve asked almost angrily.

"Dad, what are you talking about?" I chimed in.

Mom said nothing.

"I've just accepted a job at a new medical school in San Diego," Dad announced. "We're moving to California."

"What?" Steve and I just stood there, dishtowels in our hands, our mouths hanging open. We couldn't believe it. We'd had no warning that a move might be in the works. *California?* Suddenly, all thoughts of Christmas and the presents under the tree were forgotten. We were New Englanders, at home in the cold and snow, and we loved the four seasons. Now we were being told that we would have to leave our friends, the winter sports we loved, and our familiar way of life to go to *California*. We didn't know much about California—remember, we didn't have a TV—but we knew it was a lot different from New Hampshire. It was the end of the rebellious 1960s, when hippies and flower power and surfing were taking center stage in California. That was not our world.

Later, I learned more of the story. One of my dad's colleagues, a highly regarded obstetrician and research scientist named Ken Ryan, had been hired to help shape the new medical school at the University of California, San Diego (UCSD). Early in December, Dr. Ryan had invited Dad and a few other colleagues to spend two days with him to view the facilities and campus at UCSD. They were able to plan what the new reproductive biology department might look like, brainstorm what areas of research it should focus on, discuss who would be asked to join the faculty, and talk about how the school might attract other leading scientists to become one of the premier medical schools in the nation. Dad didn't know it at the time, but he was being considered as a candidate to join the faculty at UCSD. He immediately fell in love with the place and the people, so when Dr. Ryan *did* suggest that Dad consider joining him in San Diego, he was eager and ready to listen.

In my father's mind, the timing for a move was right. He felt that recent changes mandated by the dean at Dartmouth's medical school would likely dilute the quality of the students' education there. Dad also believed he had taken the pathology department as far as he could at Dartmouth and was ready for a new challenge. He was intrigued by the idea of helping to build a new, first-rate medical school with a truly extraordinary group of research scientists. As comfortable as Dad was at Dartmouth, he was getting antsy for a change.

Mom, it turned out, hadn't been too hard to convince either. Though she liked Hanover and worried about the infamous California drug scene, she had grown weary of the long New Hampshire winters. The thought of never having to shovel another walkway brought a smile to her face. Ingrid was as surprised by the news as Steve and I were, but she was caught up in the excitement and possibilities of a new environment. For Steve and me, though, the idea of moving away from all of our friends and activities in Hanover felt traumatic. Steve was in the midst of his junior year of high school and was one of New England's top junior ski racers, often beating racers who would end up on the US Olympic team. Now he would have to finish high school in unfamiliar territory, starting over for his senior year without a single friend.

My closest buddies, meanwhile, were my hockey friends. Three of us hung out together as often as we could, skating on frozen ponds or sneaking into the Dartmouth rink to get extra ice time. We loved to watch the college players practice as we walked home from school, and it was even more exciting to watch their games. Before our big games, we had developed a ritual of going to a small diner in town for lunch, always ordering the same thing, and then getting psyched to play. We talked a lot about our future hockey dreams, hoping to play somewhere together in college.

In an instant, all those dreams had come crashing down. I was devastated. I was sure there would be no hockey for me in San Diego. But there was no debate on the move—Dad and Mom had decided. Our last day in Hanover would be in June, right after the school year ended.

The next few months flew by, and before we knew it, we were packing up our belongings—including our frames of butterflies and animal skulls, which we strapped to the roof of our new station wagon—for the long drive from the northeastern corner of the United States to the southwestern tip of the country. For Steve, Ingrid, and I, pulling out of the driveway of our beloved Hanover home was truly a sad moment. The fact that we had to sell the farm made it even tougher.

The trip west included a final visit to the Catskill Game Farm and stops at the Lincoln Park Zoo in Chicago, the Denver Zoo, and Pikes Peak in Colorado's Rocky Mountains. Finally, we began seeing signs for San Diego, and we arrived at our new home.

I had to admit that our newly built house in the coastal town of La Jolla was beautiful. Unlike Hanover, however, there was hardly any room between the homes. Located on a hill above La Jolla Shores beach and part of a new subdivision, our two-story house had a tiny yard that hadn't been landscaped yet. But we could see the ocean from the second floor, at least for a couple of years until a house blocked our view. Because we were in a new neighborhood, many of the homes surrounding us were still empty. The area didn't feel warm or neighborly. To make matters worse, the moving van hadn't arrived yet and we didn't have any furniture or electricity the first night. Watching the palm trees on our hill sway in the ocean breeze was a bit surreal and reminded us that we weren't in New Hampshire anymore. I wondered what kind of life Dad was getting us into.

While the rest of us began settling into our new city, Dad was ready to get to work. His new laboratory was temporarily established in the one-year-old John Muir Biology Building on UCSD's beautiful campus, which was close enough for him to ride his bike from home. Right after he and his colleagues finished setting up their lab, the Muir College provost stopped by to meet the new arrivals. The provost turned out to be John Stewart, a former Dartmouth English professor who had once lived with his family near us in Hanover but had moved before we got to know them. Dad and Provost Stewart enjoyed reminiscing about Dartmouth and discussing people they each knew. I was happy to learn he had a son who would be going into the 10th grade like me.

My father's new research colleagues were among the best and brightest in the nation. His lab neighbor was John Holland, who would become a pioneer in virology and the study of ribonucleic acid. Down the hall was Gordon Sato, a cell biologist who would identify the protein growth factors that allowed mammalian cells to grow in tissue cultures. Other regular research partners included UCSD's Sam Yen, who would become a leading figure in reproductive endocrinology, and neuroscientist Roger Guillemin of the Salk Institute for Biological Studies. Guillemin was considered the founder of neuroendocrinology, and his study of brain hormones led to treatments for disorders ranging from infertility to pituitary tumors. He would be awarded the Nobel Prize in 1977.

This team of exceptional scientists began learning how to perform a radioimmunoassay (RIA), a new and more precise technique for measuring hormone levels in the blood. Using the RIA method, they began a systematic study of steroids and other hormones in women. Roger Guillemin was in the process of discovering gonadotropin-releasing hormone (GnRH), which causes the brain's pituitary gland to make and secrete hormones that trigger the production of testosterone in men and estrogen and progesterone in women. As an experiment, Dad injected the hormone into Roger Guillemin and Sam Yen (with their permission, of course)! The team's work led to advancements in the medical treatment of infertility and prostate cancer.

In addition to his ongoing research, Dad taught classes at UCSD's medical school and performed regular examinations of interesting placentas sent to him from across the county. It wasn't long before hospital pathologists from all over San Diego began calling him whenever a baby born with congenital malformations had died. Dad would perform the autopsy and examine the placenta to learn what he could to prevent similar birth defects in the future.

Ken Jones, who had just joined the university faculty as an assistant professor in 1974, became a partner in this endeavor. "I would drive out to the hospital, pick up a body, put it in the back of my Volkswagen Bug—which of course you could never do today—and drive it to the morgue so Kurt could perform the autopsy," he remembers. "I would then peer over his shoulder as he worked to see what I could learn."

At UCSD, Dr. Jones would become a world-renowned pediatrician and researcher in the field of birth defects as well as one of Dad's most important colleagues and friends. Over the next few decades, they would publish many articles together detailing their exciting discoveries.

Dad hosted a weekly perinatal pathology conference at UCSD for students and faculty at 9:15 a.m. every Wednesday in the morgue of the university's medical center in Hillcrest, a community in San Diego. According to Ken Jones, the 45-minute conferences were an invaluable learning experience. The conferences were open to anybody who wanted to expand their understanding.

"I always said it was the best conference I attended all year, and I got the chance to do it *every* week," says Dr. Jones. "Kurt would present the pathology of an abnormal placenta and then start calling on people to comment on everything, including how it might've affected the babies. It was amazing to be part of, because of Kurt and his extensive knowledge. He had a deep knowledge of human biology and reproduction and what led to problems in fetal development, along with an incredible understanding of maternal physiology, the physiology of pregnancy, and the physiology and development of the fetal placenta. It was basically the entire perinatal spectrum. What also made it special was his engaging personality. He was bigger than life."

Dr. Jones got to know my dad well during their 45 years of collaboration and friendship. He admired Dad's character and observed firsthand his passion and driven nature.

"I will never forget the first day I walked into Kurt's office," Dr. Jones recalls. "On his desk was a plaque that read, 'Is Integrity Extinct?' He cared very much about integrity. He also challenged people if he thought they were looking at things in ways that he didn't agree. He did this in order to stimulate a conversation and debate."

According to Dr. Jones, Dad was sometimes abrupt. When the phone on his desk rang, he picked it up and barked, "This is Benirschke. What do you want?"

"That's what Kurt was about," Dr. Jones says. "He didn't like to mess around with niceties and didn't want to hear excuses. His attitude was, 'Just give me the facts, tell me what's up, and I'll deal with it.'"

From Dr. Jones's point of view, it wasn't that Dad was unfeeling. He generously gave his time to people who had a sincere interest in learning and advancing science. But he had little patience for people he felt were wasting his time. There was too much to do and too much to discover.

He also had little patience for people who didn't take science as seriously as he did. Dr. Jones relates the story of an obstetrics department conference that Dad hosted—another of his regular activities. The conference was held in a relatively small room on campus, and lunch was provided for the attendees. One day, as Dad discussed slides projected on a screen, a man quietly got up and headed toward the exit.

Dad paused in midsentence. "You back there!" he called out, stopping the man dead in his tracks. "You came here today just to get lunch? You're leaving this conference before we get to the important part!" The man, not sure what to do, accelerated his exit, escaping more of my dad's wrath as he slipped out of the room.

"I don't think Kurt ever cared about what people thought of him," Dr. Jones says. "He wasn't motivated by approval or recognition. He was motivated by doing something for humanity, by increasing knowledge that he could tell the world about."

Dad certainly had new opportunities to increase his knowledge at UCSD. In no time, he was fully engulfed in life as a university research scientist and instructor. But he hadn't forgotten his passion for understanding animals and what they could teach about pathology and reproduction. His new friend, San Diego Zoo Director Charlie Schroeder, made sure of that. Soon after my father arrived in San Diego, Charlie asked if he would be willing to serve on the Zoo's newly formed research committee. Dad, of course, said yes.

Once again, our life was about to change.

CHAPTER 13

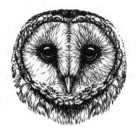

CONNECTIONS

The night was still; the only sound was the shrill chirping of crickets. In the moonlight, Dad and I lay side by side, our bellies pressed against the blanket we'd brought with us, trying hard not to make a sound. Our perch on the small hill provided a perfect view of our target, a hole on a cliff wall 30 feet away. Dad nudged me with his elbow. It was my turn to take the shot. I squinted and took aim.

We weren't snipers engaging an enemy. It was 3 a.m. on a Thursday during the spring of 1971, and we were in a deserted stretch of the San Pasqual Valley near Escondido, California, part of northern San Diego County. We were there to photograph one of my favorite birds, the barn owl. Despite knowing that in just a few hours I'd be fighting to keep my bleary eyes open during classes at La Jolla High School, I was having a blast.

It was shortly after our move to San Diego that Dad and I started making late-night excursions there. The year before, after a decade of dreams and discussions,

Charlie Schroeder and the San Diego Zoo had leased 1,800 acres of semi-arid hills, scrub brush, and cacti from the city of San Diego to establish what would become the San Diego Wild Animal Park (today the San Diego Zoo Safari Park). Charlie's vision was to create a large, beautiful environment where animals from similar regions would have space to roam and interact, where visitors could safely view wildlife in naturalistic habitats, and where animals were more likely to breed and develop self-sustaining herds. The Wild Animal Park would also advance conservation. There, researchers could study wildlife and their behaviors in a setting that was a safe haven for all, especially some of the world's most endangered species.

When Dad joined the Zoo's conservation research committee, he let the Zoo staff know he was interested in collecting samples for his research whenever they became available, including skin and placenta tissue, eggs, and sperm. As the Park was built and more animals moved in, he had more opportunities to add to his knowledge. This usually occurred when an animal was born, died, or needed to be tranquilized for a medical procedure. Staff members were trained to call Dad—even in the middle of the night—and say something like, "Dr. B, a baby antelope was just born. Do you want to come out?"

His answer was always, "Absolutely, I'll be right there." His next move was to come into my bedroom and wake me so we could be on our way.

Most high school kids wouldn't appreciate having their dad interrupt their peaceful slumber to take a middle-of-the-night drive into the hills, but I loved it. I'd throw on my jeans and grab a jacket, and in minutes we'd be racing through the dark on what used to be Route 395. It helped that we rode in Dad's pride and joy, a refurbished red 1960 Mercedes 300 SL two-seat convertible. We loved to drive to the Wild Animal Park with the top down, the wind whipping at my baseball hat and Dad's black beanie, both of us excited to see what would be at the other end of our 45-minute drive.

Dad rarely showed his emotions and wasn't the easiest guy to connect with, so I considered our adventures on these nights to be special. It was great to share our mutual passion for nature and animals—it was our thing. At the Park, I'd help him use his biopsy kit to collect a tissue sample, or I'd take pictures of whatever he was doing. During the drive there and back, I'd scour the fences and telephone poles, watching for movement or anything interesting. One night as we neared the Park on the rural, winding roads, I noticed large white birds flying off the fence posts that lined the fields.

"Dad," I said, "those white birds are barn owls! Let's see if we can follow 'em and find out where they roost or nest."

So we did. Over a succession of evening and late-night trips to the Wild Animal Park, we discovered well-used roosts for barn owls and great horned owls. Those rural roads often cut through hillocks that rose up on both sides of the pavement, and many of the owl nests were maybe 15 feet above the road in a hole in the clay of the cliffs.

Over time, we found other nests in trees and barns. Once, we followed an owl to a barn and got permission from the owner to investigate. We searched everywhere in the rafters but couldn't find the nest. Baffled, we went back the next day, and from the barn's second story, Dad and I climbed to the lip of a 10-foot-wide, empty water tank. When we pointed a flashlight beam into the tank, we saw two owl eggs and three babies that had already hatched. The owlets weren't pleased to see us. They immediately adopted a threatening posture, spreading their developing wings, showing us their sharp talons, and trying to look as big and menacing as possible. They also made a powerful, loud hissing noise that sounded like a den full of snakes, which caused Dad and me to jerk back in surprise.

My father and I became fascinated by these distinctive birds of prey. We noted the piles of bones and other material on the road beneath their roosts and nests. We learned that owls regurgitate what they can't digest in tightly compacted "pellets," usually right before they go hunting for the evening. These pellets consist of bones, small skulls, and fur from the rodents, birds, and bugs that make up owls' meals. Eager to learn more, I began collecting these pellets, taking them home, and pulling them apart to see what I might find. I was particularly interested in the skulls of the small animals the owls had ingested, because most were still fully intact and revealed the owls' varied diet. It wasn't unusual to find a rabbit skull or the skulls of small birds, kangaroo rats, and gophers, all in the same pile of pellets. As usual, Dad and I boiled the skulls to clean them. Soon we had dozens of skulls that I neatly mounted inside a glass frame display. The display still hangs on my office wall today and reminds me of those special nights.

By this time, Dad was an accomplished photographer, all self-taught. I also had an interest in photography, so he taught me the relationship between shutter speed, f-stop, and depth of field, as well as how to develop black-and-white film and print the pictures in a darkroom.

We decided we needed to apply our photography skills to our new interest in owls, so Dad purchased a 500mm telephoto lens to attach to his trusty Leica camera. We couldn't wait to capture our beloved owls on film.

On that spring night in 1971, I held the camera and zoomed in with the telephoto lens to get a better look at the barn owl nest, located in a hole on the cliff wall. I could see a pair of eggs in my viewfinder along with three tiny owlets, one larger than the others, each watching the sky and waiting for their parents to return from a hunt. I squeezed the shutter and got several shots.

In that moment, I couldn't help feeling blessed. Here I was, away from the commotion and distraction of classes, homework, and worries about the future, enjoying the still night and observing the wonders of nature firsthand. Nothing around us moved. Above us, the Milky Way stretched across the sky, the stars incredibly bright and detailed. The sense of serenity was profound. Best of all, I knew that Dad loved being here too—we were sharing the experience together.

A minute later, the faint whisper of wings interrupted the quiet night. Dad leaned my way. "Rolf, look over there. One of the parents is coming back."

We watched the barn owl, its white chest bright in the moonlight, circle the nest and land nearby. After inspecting its surroundings for a moment, it flapped its wings again and descended into the nest. Even from across the road, I could hear the owlets clicking with excitement. Through the viewfinder, I watched the adult barn owl drop a rodent from its mouth into the nest. It began to tear the rodent into pieces with its beak and feed the pieces to the owlets, which jostled for position while I snapped several more pictures. I passed the camera to Dad so he could see what was going on and take several more shots. A few minutes later, the barn owl flew off to hunt again. I grinned at Dad, and we both shook our heads. This was a night to remember!

We had many other adventures in the San Pasqual Valley. Once, our frequent stops and starts along the road to watch owls and collect their pellets attracted the attention of a county sheriff's deputy. Unbeknownst to us, he'd been following us from a distance and finally decided to investigate. He pulled us over and cautiously walked up to the side of our car. The deputy shined his light into our eyes and said, "Good evening. What are you two doing out here so late?"

Dad replied, "We're shooting owls."

"You're what?" The deputy's expression immediately turned serious.

I realized that this conversation was getting off to a bad start. "No, no, Dad," I interjected. "We're taking *pictures* of owls." I pointed to our camera. "See this lens?" I said to the deputy. "We're taking pictures. There's a nest just down the road. Do you want to see it?"

The deputy looked from Dad's face to mine and then back to Dad's, his expression softening into a smile. "Okay," he said. "I'll follow you and take a look."

We led the deputy to a spot about 40 yards away where the road cut through a hillock. Once we were out of our cars, Dad pointed to a hole on the cliff to our left that was marked by white droppings from the resident owls. "That's the nest, up there. And down here," he said, motioning at a pile of pellets, "are the animal remains they regurgitate after eating."

The deputy looked puzzled. "Okay, I see," he said. "But why are you so interested in this?"

Dad explained his connection to the Zoo and the new Wild Animal Park, which was still being built. The deputy finally seemed to accept our explanation and returned to his patrol car with a slight shake of his head. I breathed a sigh of relief. I could just imagine the look on Mom's face if she had to come and bail Dad and me out of jail for "shooting" owls!

Once I had my driver's license, Mom and Dad allowed me to bring some of my high school buddies "owling." We also drove into the desert to catch snakes and lizards that ventured onto the still-warm pavement on cool nights. We'd photograph the reptiles and then let them go. Sometimes my friends and I would camp overnight in the desert and return home the next day. It was always fun, but none of those outings compared to the times I had with Dad.

Part of what made those nights with my father so special was that he had a harder time appreciating some of my other interests—namely, sports. I'd always enjoyed athletics. For me, nothing was quite as exhilarating as passing a puck back and forth while skating at full speed on a frozen pond, or weaving past a defender on a soccer field, or racing down a mountain on skis. I was afraid that the move to San Diego had ended most of my athletic pursuits and dreams. The only sport I thought I might still be able to play was tennis. The problem was that I was small for my age. (And I do mean small—5 feet 4 inches tall and just 112 pounds at the start of my sophomore year of high school.) An ill-advised attempt at wrestling didn't improve the situation. In my first match, I was pinned in just 17 seconds. It was humiliating, but I finished out the season because the team didn't have anybody else to wrestle in the 112-pound weight class. Ugh.

Things began to look up during my junior year when a group of us transplanted

East Coasters and a few foreign exchange students got together and formed the first soccer team at La Jolla High School. This was a sport I knew and loved and could play, and I was just starting to grow into my full frame. One afternoon after soccer practice, a couple of the guys from the football team brought over a football and asked if any of us had ever kicked one. Soccer-style kicking was now all the rage in the National Football League, and they were looking for a kicker for the high school football team. Before we knew it, five of us were locked in a field goal–kicking competition. If we missed a kick, we were out of the competition. With each kick, we moved the ball out five yards farther. I'd always had a strong leg and found that kicking a football was just like making a goal kick in soccer. It was easy. When I drilled a kick from 50 yards, I was named the winner of our impromptu contest, and we all had a good laugh.

What none of us realized was that the head football coach, Gene Edwards, was watching from beside the gym. After seeing what I had done, Coach Edwards called me over and asked if I would be interested in kicking for the high school team next season, my senior year. It took some convincing, but I eventually agreed to give it a try. It turned out to be not that difficult, and I ended up making 12 of 14 field goal attempts and being named to the San Diego Section's All-California Interscholastic Federation first team.

It was fun to play well and contribute to the team, but my success in football made little impression on Dad. To him, athletics was at best a form of exercise and at worst a distraction from more important matters. He was busy teaching at the UC San Diego School of Medicine, volunteering on the Zoo's research committee, and speaking around the country. He never made it to any of my high school football or soccer games, so when college football coaches began calling from Stanford, USC, San Diego State, and the University of California, Berkeley, Dad was more amused than anything else. The real world, he told me, wasn't about kicking a football around on Saturday afternoons. Dad believed that I should go to college for an education in science, not sports. I agreed, but I wouldn't have minded if he had shown just a little more interest in my athletic pursuits.

Dad was more than happy, however, to encourage my interest in wildlife. When I graduated from La Jolla High School in 1973, he surprised me with an unusual graduation gift—the chance to spend three weeks at Ian Player's Wilderness Leadership School with five other international students, living and studying in game reserves outside Durban, South Africa. The experience had a profound impact on me as an 18-year-old, increasing my appreciation for the fauna and flora of our world. When the wilderness school ended, I extended my stay and spent several more weeks in South Africa at the Umfolozi Game Reserve, where I was able to help with a project to capture and return critically endangered white rhinos to repopulate their original breeding areas.

The trip affirmed that I'd made the right choice in deciding to study zoology. I'd selected the best school for zoology on the West Coast, the University of California, Davis (UC Davis). Dad had been pleased, and I enrolled in the fall of 1973.

I had no idea if Davis had a football team and didn't give it much thought when I showed up for school. As far as I was concerned, my short-lived football career was over, and I was now focused on my studies. But a week after school started, I got a call from the head football coach at Davis, Jim Sochor. Somehow, Jim had heard that I had kicked in high school with some success. Despite my reservations, he talked me into coming out and kicking for the freshman team. That went well enough that I was in line to be the varsity kicker the next year. By then, however, I'd made some good friends on the soccer team and found that I really missed the fast-paced action of that sport. In college, football and soccer were both played in the fall, which meant I had to choose one or the other—at least I thought. But Jim Sochor worked with the soccer coach and the athletic director to come up with a plan to "share" me for the season if I was willing to give it a try.

When I explained all this to Dad, he was skeptical but said he was willing to support me as long as I kept up my studies. I then went to my best buddies on both the soccer and football teams and asked if they were okay with me splitting my time. Once they assured me that they were, I was all in and ended up playing both sports for the rest of my time at Davis. Dad never did see me play either sport at Davis—but I know he was proud when I earned my zoology degree, graduating in 1977.

I decided to continue my education after college. I had been accepted to several graduate school programs and was trying to decide which one to pick as my senior year wound down. At the same time, I'd received lots of letters from NFL and Canadian Football League teams suggesting that I was good enough for the pros, but I'd decided that they probably sent those letters to most senior athletes. Then, to my surprise, the defending Super Bowl champions, the Oakland Raiders, chose me in the NFL draft. I was sitting in class when my roommate snuck in, interrupted the lecture, and told me the Raiders had called. I was the second-to-last player taken in the 12th and final round.

My selection surprised Dad even more. He was at work on the day of the draft when a medical colleague from Boston called and said, "Congratulations, K. B., on your son getting drafted!" (Dad's close colleagues and friends often called him "K. B.")

"What?" Dad said, not understanding. "Drafted? I thought the draft ended years ago!" He was thinking of the military draft, of course. Since he didn't follow football, he had no clue that his friend was talking about the NFL draft.

Being selected by the Raiders gave me something to think about. I reasoned that the chance to try to play pro football was a once-in-a-lifetime opportunity. After a lot of soul-searching and talks with my friends, I decided to give it a try. I figured if I didn't make the final roster, I could always go back to graduate school with some good stories. But I knew I would never have another chance to see what pro football was all about.

Not surprisingly, my dad didn't understand my decision. He felt I was wasting time that could be better spent advancing my career. But for me, it was an important step toward making my own choices and taking responsibility for my own life.

⁂

My older brother, Steve, found his own ways of connecting with Dad. One of those was through their mutual love of cars. Dad had admired the Mercedes brand since he was a kid and bought a used 1960 300 SL roadster in 1971 with a little extra money made from finally selling our house in Hanover. The car needed work, so he and Steve plunged in, doing repairs on weekends and often late into the evening on weeknights. They started with the engine. Then they added chrome plating to the bumpers and trim and redid the electrical system. Next, the car needed a new paint job—which they learned to do themselves after buying a compressor and spray gun. They replaced the headlights, the hard top, and many parts that they found in junkyards. They even tracked down the original leather luggage that came with the car, obtained from a fellow member of the Mercedes classic car club.

They did such a good job restoring the 300 SL that it eventually became a show vehicle, one that Dad took to car shows on weekends but still drove to work during the week. Soon Steve also bought his own classic sports car. He found a used Mercedes 190 SL designed along the same lines as the 300 SL, only smaller. Steve's vehicle needed even more refurbishing than Dad's car. He and Dad made friends with junkyard owners, other car enthusiasts, and car specialists in the area. There were many weeks when the two of them spent more time in the garage than they did in the house.

Refurbishing cars wasn't their only shared passion. Like Dad, Steve developed a love of medicine. After graduating from high school, he enrolled in the biology premed program at UCSD. He lived at home while attending college, which allowed him to continue to work on cars with Dad when he had time, before graduating in 1975. Steve decided on Case Western Reserve University in Cleveland to begin his medical studies.

Of the three siblings, Ingrid probably had the hardest time connecting with Dad. Like Steve and me, she also enjoyed sports, including figure skating, volleyball, and soccer. She was a very good student and developed a particular interest in languages, taking French and German in Hanover and again at La Jolla High School. She attended college at UCSD for two years before studying abroad for one year each in France and Germany. "That was the best decision of my life," she recalls now. "It was a great experience. I learned more in those two years abroad than I could have anywhere else, and I became fluent in French and German."

Ingrid graduated after another quarter at UCSD, but she had no idea what to do next. She considered learning Spanish and going into social work, but Dad had other ideas. "You should try publishing," he said. "You have a gift with words, and you know science. Why don't you talk to someone at Springer, my publisher?"

So, on a family trip to the East Coast, Ingrid interviewed with a social worker and then with a representative at Springer-Verlag, the company that had published several of Dad's books. The latter meeting eventually led to a second interview, a job offer, a quick decision to move to Manhattan, and a 30-year career in publishing.

"I have to give Dad credit," Ingrid says today with a smile. "He was absolutely right. Publishing was the perfect career for me for so many reasons, including the chance to use my German and French. I'm really glad that I listened to him."

"Dad had so many great qualities," Ingrid adds. "I'm truly grateful for both of my parents. But I do wish that while I was growing up, I could have shared more about the things *I* was excited about with Dad."

As intensely curious as Dad was about science, animals, and the world at large, he seemed to find it difficult to devote that same energy to his kids' interests when they didn't match his own. If you were a member of the Benirschke family, you saw this play out at dinner. Mom always prepared a great meal—she was a wonderful cook—and we'd all sit down at the dining table every night, with Dad at the head. As soon as we were served, he would launch into a description of his day—the exciting research he was doing, the discoveries he'd made or was on the brink of making, the next experiment he hoped to conduct. When he finished eating, he would excuse himself and head off to his study to smoke a pipe and read or work. His stories and updates were always interesting and often fascinating, but I don't think it ever occurred to Dad to ask about what the rest of us were doing.

One night when I was home from college for a quick visit, I got frustrated with him. We were all at the table for dinner, and, as usual, Dad dominated the conversation. At the end of the meal, he finished speaking and got up to leave the room. "Wait a minute, Dad," I said, speaking to him a bit more forcefully than I ever had. "Sit down, please. Tonight, I want to tell you about *my* day and what *I'm* doing."

I wasn't sure how he would react. He looked startled for a moment and then said, "Just a minute." He walked upstairs, then returned carrying a pipe and tobacco pouch. He filled the pipe, placed it in his mouth, leaned back, and said, "All right. Talk."

I don't even remember what I said after that, but it was nice to know that for at least one evening, I had my father's full attention.

Although Dad may not have been outwardly interested in every aspect of his kids' lives, he still found ways to show that he cared. When we were young and he was home, he was actively involved, giving us evening baths, changing diapers, taking us skiing or skating, and spending time with us in lots of different ways. When he traveled to give talks or visit other scientists, he always sent postcards from wherever he was, and he went out of his way to include the whole family on many trips that created great memories for all of us.

Dad wasn't what you'd call a gifted encourager, but he had his moments.

Ingrid recalls that when we still lived in Hanover—she was probably 11 or 12—she went through a phase where she was afraid of the dark. During that time, she couldn't relax enough to fall asleep unless she crawled into bed with Mom and Dad. On one of those evenings when Ingrid showed up in the middle of the night, Dad gently walked her back into her bedroom and sat on the bed with her.

"Ingrid, there are nights when I can't sleep either," he said. "You know what I do? I turn on the light and read for a while. I just embrace it."

His calm words were exactly what Ingrid needed to hear. After that, she got up on restless nights, sat in a rocking chair, and read a book or listened to a record by one of her favorite singers, Petula Clark. After a little while, she found she was ready to go back to sleep. Knowing that Dad had the same issue and learned how to handle it took the fear away for Ingrid.

Dad cared about what kind of people we were, and he expected us to be polite, grateful, and good citizens of the world. To that end, he often quoted phrases (usually in German) that were important to him—lessons that he wanted us to remember. One of those sayings can be roughly translated, "The way that you call into the forest will return to you." In other words, the way we approach the world will be reflected back to us. Dad showed us the truth of those words by the way he lived. People responded positively to his upbeat, optimistic, enthusiastic manner and passion. Someone once said that he could charm the birds from the trees—people *wanted* to partner with him and help him. His positive, can-do attitude was a huge reason for his achievements and success, and it was a model for Steve, Ingrid, and me.

Over time, we began to appreciate more and more what an amazing man Dad was and how he helped shape the people we've become. His integrity, work ethic, generosity, and desire to make the world a better place were just a few of his outstanding qualities.

Of course, our mother represented the other half of the equation that made our family work. We were incredibly blessed to have Mom. It seemed that she was always there to fill in whatever gaps Dad had as a parent. She showered us with affection, validation, approval, and encouragement, without any judgment. She listened patiently and with great interest when we had exciting news to share or a problem we needed to talk about.

One day in Hanover, I lost an important ski race to Steve. Both of us were competitive and hated to lose. I was upset because I felt I should have won, and I aired my frustration to Mom. She said, gently, "Well, Rolf, you have to learn how to lose as well as how to win." Her words put the situation in perspective. At the time, it was exactly what I needed to hear. That was Mom. She always knew just what to say.

Dad was the leader of our family, pointing the way forward and showing us how to live a meaningful life, but Mom was the glue that held us all together. It wasn't always easy, and our parents weren't perfect—no parents are—but in different ways, they showed their love and devotion to us countless times, gave us a secure home to grow up in, and encouraged us to make a difference. For that and for them, we will always be grateful.

CHAPTER 14

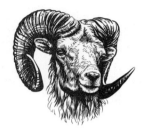

A Vision and a Leader

When Charlie Schroeder invited Dad to join the San Diego Zoo's research committee in 1970, active zoo research was still a rare phenomenon worldwide. The vast majority of zoos focused their time and budgets on creating an interesting and interactive experience for the public and maintaining a healthy animal population. For most zoological institutions, conducting long-term, rigorous scientific research that could lead to a better understanding of animals and conservation was much lower on the priority list—if it was done at all.

In San Diego, the research committee's early efforts mostly consisted of reviewing requests from outside scientists for tissue samples and getting access to the Zoo's animals. This did not satisfy my father, of course. As he bluntly put it to the committee, "I don't have time to come to a meeting once a month just to have a glass of wine. If we're going to have this committee, we're going to *do* something and we're going to *be* something."

It wasn't long before Dad was chosen to chair the research committee. He decided that the committee members should first tour the Zoo and identify specific problems that research might solve. Their initial stop was at the habitat for the greater one-horned rhinoceros. In a conversation with the rhinoceros care specialist, Dad asked why the rhinos weren't breeding.

"Well, Doc, we imported this female rhino from India at a cost of $20,000," the wildlife care specialist said. "The male is trying to mate all right, but as soon as he does, he pushes the female into the ditch that separates the habitat from the visitors. Then I have to get a crane to lift her out of the ditch and return her to the habitat. This has happened over and over, and the crane is getting too expensive to lease . . . to say nothing about their inability to get together to mate!"

As a result of this meeting, Dad and the committee recommended that the rhinos be transferred to the new Wild Animal Park, which had just opened to the public. In this environment with lots of open space, the rhinos had no trouble mating, and they started to reproduce.

It had taken only a little "research" to solve the problem—merely an on-site visit and a conversation. Imagine, Dad and others thought, what a dedicated conservation research group could do! He next challenged the committee to present a plan to the Zoo's board of trustees to show how they could establish and support research on an ongoing basis at the Zoo.

With the help of other committee members, Dad wrote two white papers outlining the case for a funded conservation research division within the Zoological Society of San Diego (now San Diego Zoo Wildlife Alliance), which oversaw all of the Zoo's activities and departments. In 1974, the board considered the formal proposal at a special meeting. The proposal included the statement, "We believe that the possibility now exists for our Zoo to become the world leader in this field, as it has in exhibition and is evolving to be in conservation. We believe that the idea is viable and represents one of the most important and necessary next steps in the development of the Zoo."

Though a few board members expressed reservations, the proposal had the support of the recently retired director, Charlie Schroeder, and the new Zoo director, Charles "Chuck" Bieler. The motion passed to establish a conservation research branch with an initial budget of $300,000.

Chuck Bieler was charged with hiring a director for the new effort. He did not have to look far. "I like to deal with people I know," Chuck explains now, "and I knew that Kurt had the vision and energy to do this. I'd heard his vision at the committee meetings, and I had experienced his passion. He had a message: 'We are consumers of wildlife. What we've got to do is become providers of wildlife. We've got to save and perpetuate what we have here, and we've got to get veterinary medicine to the place where human medicine is today.'"

Chuck met with Dad in the director's office. "Dr. Benirschke, you got me into this hole," he said, applying a measure of good-natured guilt. "I believe in what we want to do, but now we need a director. It's got to be the right person, not someone who will come in and play a game of politics. We need someone with a vision. Would you be interested?"

My father considered the offer for a moment. "I might be," he said. "Would you allow me to continue to work at the university as well?"

"I'm amenable to looking at and discussing anything you come up with," Chuck answered.

In those few seconds, Dad had already made up his mind. "All right," he said. "I'll work one day a week at the university and four days at the Zoo."

Chuck knew then that he had his director *and* that he'd made a bargain in the process. "When Kurt said one day at the university and four at the Zoo," Chuck says, "I knew that really meant five days a week at the university and seven days at the Zoo. That's just how Kurt was."

Though the effort was initially described as the Zoo's new research department, a more formal name emerged—the Center for Research on Endangered Species (CRES). Since animal research was controversial in some quarters, the board decided later to change the name to the Center for Reproduction of Endangered Species.

By late 1974, the new venture had acquired a vision, a budget, and a leader. Dad's next step was to hire a staff capable of achieving his ambitious plans.

∞

"The first time I met Kurt Benirschke was at his university office for an interview," recalls one of my father's longtime employees. "His face was black and blue, and his arm was in a cast. He'd cut the cast apart and wrapped it with tape because he thought it was too tight. Apparently, he'd been painting his house a couple of weeks earlier, had unwisely put a ladder on top of a table to reach the higher parts of an outside wall, and had fallen and broken his arm. He was a mess."

The interviewee was a native New Yorker named Mary Byrd (now Mary Cole), who was applying to be Dad's secretary at the new conservation research center. Her knowledge of animals was limited, she admitted, to dogs, cats, and hamsters, but she'd been to nursing school and she needed a job.

"You don't know anything about animals, and you can hardly type," Dad said. "What makes you think you can do this?"

"That's true," Mary said. "But let me tell you something. I promise you I'll do anything anyone else can, but I'll always do it better." That confidence and can-do attitude matched Dad's, and that was what he liked to hear. Though many of the 65 applicants had better credentials, Mary got the job, and she and my dad forged a special relationship.

It didn't take long for him to test Mary's promise. On one of their first days together, he handed her a stack of papers, each with the title of a different animal, but with only the animal's scientific name. "Put these where they belong," Dad said before heading out the door.

"I had no idea what I was looking at or where the papers should go,"

Mary remembers today. When another staff member walked by the office, she stopped him and asked, "Could you help me, please?" Mary explained the situation, and the staffer returned a minute later with a copy of *Walker's Mammals of the World*. "I learned the 19 orders of mammals that day, and I filed the papers," Mary says with a smile. "Later, K. B. came back to the office and asked me, 'Did you get those papers put away?' He knew darn well that when he'd left, I had no earthly idea how to file them. I just answered, 'Yes.' He didn't say another word."

But Dad hadn't finished testing Mary. A day or two later, he walked up to her desk and handed her a syringe and needle. "Go down to the reptile house and give that big iguana a shot, would you please?" he said. Once again, he was out the door before Mary could reply.

Mary had no idea how to administer a shot to a reptile, so she tracked down a veterinary intern in the building and enlisted her help. When Dad returned to the office, he asked, "You give that shot to the iguana?"

"Yes, sir," was Mary's response. As before, he said nothing more.

"It was trial by fire, you could say," Mary recalls with a smile. "But after that, everything was fine." She would become his invaluable right hand at the Zoo, helping "enormously," as Dad later wrote, "in running the place and cementing relations with the community and looking after the peace of the 'Zoo family.'"

The fledgling team also included a pair of lab technicians, Mark Bogart and Arlene Kumamoto. Mark, a UCSD graduate, would become a vital contributor to early research efforts at the Zoo before becoming the Zoo's curator of primates in the late 1970s. Later, he would earn his PhD and join a cytogenetics research group at UCSD.

Arlene became an integral member of the department—a respected favorite of Dad's and everyone she worked with. She earned her undergraduate degree in biology from UCSD in 1974 and began working for Dad in the university's lab. She became a technician for the Zoo and then a lab manager and cytogenetics specialist, which reflected her expertise in cell culture and karyotyping. In the years ahead, she would be recognized as an international authority on animal cytogenetics. To her colleagues, Arlene was known for her kindness and empathy—as well as for her fiery temper before she'd had her morning coffee.

Another key figure in those early days was Bill Lasley. Bill was conducting postdoctoral research on reproductive endocrinology at UCSD after earning his doctorate in physiology at UC Davis. Dad knew that Bill was a top-notch researcher and recruited him to pursue reproductive endocrinology at the Zoo. The timing was perfect, since Bill wasn't sure of his next career step.

"I was lucky to be in that founding group," Bill recalls. "It was the start of something really special. Kurt said we were going to do top-notch science, and we did. He built a new concept of zoo research from scratch, as good as any in the world."

Bill showed his commitment to the Zoo's new research effort by working there seven days a week while finishing his postdoctoral research at the university hospital during once-a-week all-nighters. "Kurt never questioned my hours because he was doing the same thing—burning both ends of the candle, except at a much higher level," Bill says. "He was the epitome of the saying, 'Do what you love, and you'll love what you do and make a good living at it.' He was such a good example. In a word, he was inspirational." In fact, Dad inspired Bill to help fill an important niche in the zoo world. Bill began developing new technologies and made significant contributions to the breeding and conservation of wildlife at the Zoo and at UC Davis. His research with animals eventually led to recognizing the various changes that occur as healthy women age, as well as understanding environmental hazards to human reproductive health.

Dad also helped inspire the career of another scientist who would become a central figure in the Zoo's conservation research efforts and one of his closest colleagues. In 1974, Oliver "Ollie" Ryder was finishing his PhD in biology at UCSD. "I was a graduate student living in a little house in a tiny community east of Del Mar," Ollie recalls. "I'd had an awakening about the natural world just because I started to look out the window. What bird is that? What are those native plants? I found out I was seeing rare species. It got me interested in endangered wildlife, but I had no idea how to approach that as a scientist."

At the time, most researchers didn't consider wildlife conservation a legitimate field for academic study. But Ollie knew that my father was a respected physician and scientist, so he went to Dad's office and introduced himself.

"Can a molecular biologist do anything to help save endangered species?" Ollie asked.

"Yes," Dad said. "But you're going to have to figure it out."

By the end of their conversation, he had made Ollie a life-changing offer: "If you want to work with me, you can."

"For me, that was a wonderful and enormously significant conversation and invitation," Ollie says. "That's what I've done my whole career since—to help save endangered species—and he made it possible." Dad introduced Ollie to colleagues at UC Davis who said he would have to start an entirely new field of study—what today might be termed "conservation genetics." They also encouraged him by saying, "If you can work with Benirschke, you should."

In 1975, Dad invited Ollie to join the team full-time. Over nearly 50 years (and counting), Ollie would conduct and contribute to key studies benefiting the conservation management of gorillas, California condors, black rhinos, Przewalski's horses, Anegada iguanas, bighorn sheep, and other species. As of 2022, he still serves with San Diego Zoo Wildlife Alliance as the Kleberg Endowed Director of Conservation Genetics, where he focuses his work on reducing extinction risk and contributing to wildlife recovery and the development of sustainable populations.

When Ollie joined the team, the prevailing atmosphere was one of "excitement and tension and possibility, of urgency to get things started," he explains. It was an attitude he attributed to my father. In Dad, Ollie had found a mentor who would influence and be an example to him for the rest of his career. In addition to filling that role, Dad served as something of a father figure to Ollie. "He was just so generous and encouraging with me," Ollie says. "I realize now how much he cared for me. I wouldn't be who I am and where I am today without that generosity. He took the time to encourage me. I will be forever grateful."

Nancy Czekala was another important addition to the team. Nancy had been hired at UCSD in 1970 to perform radioimmunoassays (RIAs) for Dr. Sam Yen. She also worked with Dad, taking blood samples of Zoo animals that he provided to do estrogen or testosterone analysis. One day at UCSD, Nancy went to his office and asked if he could help her come up with a project that was a class requirement for her application to veterinary school. Dad smiled and said, "Well, let's see what I have in my desk drawer." He proceeded to pull out two jars, each containing a bat embryo from the same mother. "I think we should study these," he said. Nancy's first scientific paper, published with Dad in 1974, explored why twin embryos from an African long-tongued fruit bat were different sizes.

"It was very exciting," Nancy remembers. "I learned a lot about embryology, and I learned that Kurt Benirschke was an extremely good teacher and mentor. I also learned to never, ever look in his desk drawers, unless you wanted a surprise! The things he had in there were . . . unusual."

In 1976, Nancy successfully petitioned Dad to hire her, and she joined Bill Lasley in his endocrinology work. "This ultimately led to the start of a new field of science—noninvasive endocrine monitoring of exotic wildlife. It was an amazing opportunity for me," Nancy says. She went on to publish more than 100 papers exploring reproductive changes in zoo and wild animals. Nancy and Bill were the first to develop and publish these kinds of studies, and now there is an international society of scientists who work in this field. As of 2022, Nancy is the founder and director of the Papoose Conservation Wildlife Foundation.

Over the years, many more outstanding researchers, scientists, veterinarians, students, and other professionals passed through the department and contributed to the Zoo's conservation research, creating a model that zoos across the country and around the world have emulated. Today, the Zoo's conservation department and its field programs help provide a future for rare and endangered wildlife worldwide. Yet on the day that the department was officially launched—January 1, 1975—this far-reaching future was little more than a dream in Dad's mind. It started with some skepticism, a challenge, and a large flightless bird native to South America called the Darwin's rhea.

CHAPTER 15

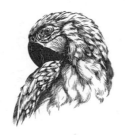

GIVE ME A PROBLEM

"Well, Professor-Doctor Benirschke, what are you going to do for me?"

It was 9 a.m. on Thursday, January 2, 1975, and my father was attending his first official meeting as director of the Zoo's new research department. He and his small team had used the winter holidays to move lab equipment and office supplies into their new quarters, a two-story, 8,000-square-foot Scripps veterinary hospital building on the Zoo grounds that had been constructed in the 1920s. They were ready to go to work.

The bespectacled gentleman attempting to provoke Dad from across the table that Thursday morning was Kenton "K. C." Lint, then curator of birds and a legend at the San Diego Zoo. K. C. had joined the Zoo as an assistant curator in 1936. Almost 40 years later, he was a widely respected pioneer who had set more than 400 records for breeding birds. He was also, like a few others on the Zoo staff, skeptical about welcoming a medical doctor into the Zoo's operations.

Dad did not shy away from the challenge. "Tell me, Mr. Lint," he said.

"What is your biggest problem?"

"What do you mean, what's my biggest problem?"

Dad leaned forward in his chair. "Give me a problem that you have," he said. "We'll take a look at it and see if we can help you figure it out."

K. C. was taken aback. "Well, can I come back to you next week on that?" he asked.

"Of course," Dad said.

The following Thursday, K. C. gave the research team its first opportunity to prove its value. The Zoo had a collection of Darwin's rheas, flightless birds that in adulthood stand about three feet high and weigh approximately 40 pounds. Despite his past success with breeding, K. C. was having trouble with the rheas. The hatchlings had a salmonella infection, and most of them were dying.

Dad and his team decided to tackle the problem by first raising the Darwin's rhea chicks in the Scripps building to get a closer look at what was happening. They decided to "paint" the rhea eggs with antibiotics to prevent any infection from penetrating the shell. Next, they had to figure out what and how to feed the newly hatched rheas. Always creative, Dad decided to borrow Mom's meat grinder to create pellet-sized portions of food. Unfortunately, this resulted in the young birds overeating. Their excessive weight gain caused the chicks to develop bent legs and clubbed feet that had to be splinted. Eventually, however, the team was successful in eliminating the salmonella infection *and* finding the right balance of food for the chicks. This was important in ensuring not only the well-being of the rheas but also the satisfaction of K. C. Lint! Dad and his team had overcome the first hurdle in gaining acceptance and respect from the Zoo staff.

Another early challenge had much wider implications. Zoo officials in San Diego and around the world were realizing that it would be increasingly difficult to import animals from the wilderness to replace individuals that had died at zoos. Wildlife habitats were shrinking, and wildlife species were becoming endangered. Countries were also increasingly hesitant to part with their animals, which they had begun to view as an asset. Zoos needed to get better at understanding their wildlife and learning how to feed their animals properly, keep them healthy, and breed them successfully. Breeding was not always easy, though. In some birds, such as parrots, it was nearly impossible to determine an individual's sex using any of the common methods like size, plumage variation, or differentiation in markings. As a result, it was hard to pair certain birds, so most zoos simply put a bunch of birds together with some nesting material and let them figure it out.

Dad discussed this challenge with endocrinologist Bill Lasley and the rest of the team. "Let's think about it," he said, "and figure out how we might apply some of the techniques we use in humans to solve this problem."

Bill proposed checking the estrogen and testosterone hormone levels in each bird's urine to determine the sex of the individual. There was one hitch, though: since parrots and other birds simultaneously excrete waste and urine from the same passage (the cloaca), collecting urine samples wouldn't be that easy. In addition, nobody had ever done this research or knew what the birds' actual hormone levels should be. To solve the problem, the researchers decided to separate the parrots, collect each bird's excrement, and measure the ratio of testosterone to estrogen. This method, called fecal steroid analysis, allowed researchers to identify the parrots with a high testosterone ratio as male and those with a high estrogen ratio as female.

This relatively simple but effective technique for determining the sex of the parrot without handling the animal had an enormous impact on breeding birds and was incorporated by zoos and breeders worldwide. In 1978, Bill was honored with a prestigious Rolex Award for Enterprise for this discovery. Dad and other members of the staff and board of trustees flew with Bill to Geneva to celebrate. Bill Lasley's discovery considerably raised the profile and stature of the Zoo's research efforts. By 1979, his method for identifying the sex of birds had grown so successful that zoos and bird breeders from around the world were sending samples to the San Diego Zoo for analysis. It wasn't long before the Zoo's research center had processed more than 1,000 samples and changed avian reproduction forever.

Another early challenge that Dad's team tackled was dolphin breeding. Most of the world's aquaria and marine animal parks, including San Diego's SeaWorld, periodically imported dolphins from their native habitat to maintain their populations. In the 1960s and 1970s, little was known about the reproduction of dolphins, and they did not consistently breed well at parks or aquariums. Dad and others decided that the answer was to collaborate, so in 1975, the Zoo hosted an international conference on dolphin biology. The conference was so well attended and so successful in encouraging scientists to share information and research that soon aquaria and marine parks had learned how to effectively breed dolphins. As a college student at the time, I even joined this research effort myself. With Dad, I published my first scientific paper, which explored the question of whether dolphins breed by spontaneous ovulation or reflex ovulation.

Buoyed by their success, Dad and his team helped organize and host an international symposium on diseases of zoo animals. This further raised the profile of the Zoo's research department and inspired research fellows from many countries to visit the San Diego Zoo. Organizations like the National Institutes of Health, the National Science Foundation, and the Scripps Research Institute recognized the research team's important advances, and they began providing grants that supported the work and hiring of additional staff. In just a few years, the number of people working at the Zoo's research center grew from a handful to more than 50. Generous donations also enabled the construction of a new, 10,000-square-foot, state-of-the-art veterinary hospital at the Zoo, and the Jennings Center for Zoological Medicine was formally dedicated on September 10, 1977.

By this time, it seemed everyone was publishing and contributing to a greater understanding of animals and reproduction. Perhaps they were driven by one of Dad's strongest beliefs: "Concepts not shared in print are concepts that do not exist." Meanwhile, and just as importantly, the Zoo's veterinarians, pathologists, and researchers were cooperating and collaborating—with both their ideas and equipment—at levels never seen before. My father and his team were hitting their stride.

Publishing, critical thinking, and hard work were Dad's standards for the research department. At the same time, his legendary impatience was also increasingly on display. When he and Bill Lasley realized one day that Bill needed more space for his endocrine laboratory, Dad could not wait for the Zoo's facilities department to process all the red tape associated with new construction. Instead, he and Bill decided to go into the lab one weekend and do the construction themselves. Bill denies that any walls were added or removed. But the following Monday, the research staff came into the office and couldn't help noticing there was now a solid wall where there had previously been a door. When word got back to the Zoo's facilities staff, they complained loudly about this encroachment on their territory. Dad and Bill survived the incident—but they were given a strong warning not to take on any more future "improvements" themselves.

Despite the high expectations within the department, the atmosphere was friendly and cooperative. Nearly every day began with my dad bursting through the double-door entrance to the Scripps building and bounding up the grand staircase next to the front desk, loudly and gleefully calling, "Ollie? Ollie?" Ollie Ryder's office was on the second floor. Several students—and a few parrots that lived in the building—learned to mimic the morning "Ollie" call. It was, according to one staff member, "sincere, irritating, and precious," all at the same time.

One tradition that Dad instituted was having the staff gather around a big table upstairs each afternoon for tea. During this break, people shared what they were working on, their progress, any needs or concerns they might have, and what they were learning from various projects. "It was wonderful," says Nancy

Czekala. "I remember it as a very kind and enriching time."

In 1976, Dad was asked to take on additional responsibilities at UCSD as the chair of the pathology department, a position he would hold for the next three years. His duties at the university meant that on Wednesdays he didn't arrive for work at the Zoo until later in the day. On one occasion, Mary (Byrd) Cole and the rest of the staff put together a humorous video entitled, "Any Wednesday." It showed what the staff was purportedly up to while Dad was away—sunbathing, reading novels, playing the accordion and video games, but then diving into what looked like a frenzy of work activity once his green Volkswagen Beetle was spotted approaching the building. Dad loved it.

Although the team found ways to add levity to their work, their focus always remained on the science. It was in those moments of learning and discovery that his colleagues most fondly remember Dad.

"I spent hours on the two-headed microscope with K. B.," Bill Lasley recalls. "Sometimes it was my slide, sometimes his, but always there was a tutorial at the most academic yet somehow still personal level. I was sitting less than a foot away from the master and trying to absorb what I could of his constant narrative. He always removed the mechanical slide mounts on the slide stage and used only his fingers to move the slide into various positions. Inevitably, I would bump my side of the scope, which was connected to his, causing an uncomfortable jolt to his eyepiece. Despite my clumsiness, he never once complained. Instead, with just a slight grunt of annoyance, he kept right on with the lesson. I'm sure most, perhaps all, of K. B.'s fellows, students, and colleagues would remember him best in this way. It was, somehow, the best of times."

I know firsthand what it was like to be in the department in those early days. As a college student, I worked at the Zoo in the summer of 1974 and then at the research center the next two summers. It was fascinating to be in an environment full of bright, curious, enthusiastic people who were all doing something important. Now, when Dad talked about his day at the dinner table, I had a much better understanding of what he and his colleagues faced and how important the work was. It was amazing to be around so many different animals up close and to learn about some of the challenges they encountered. I loved being able to walk around the Zoo during short breaks or on my way to one of my tasks. I reveled in the beauty and diversity of so much wildlife, hoping that one day I could see these animals in their natural habitat.

During those summers, I assisted wherever I was needed, including with the Darwin's rhea project and with Bill Lasley's efforts to identify the sex of parrots. I also helped Ollie Ryder with a project involving the Zoo's Galápagos tortoises. The tortoises came from several of the different islands within Ecuador's Galápagos Islands archipelago, and we wondered if the tortoises had become separate species, like the famous finches that Charles Darwin first wrote about when he described the process of evolution.

Some tortoises looked quite different from the others, with markedly different shells and neck lengths. One tortoise had a shell with a saddle curve that allowed it to stretch out and maneuver its long neck more easily than the others. This adaptation, which had occurred over many generations, allowed it to eat low-hanging fruit from trees that were found only on the island where it lived. Ollie and I hoped to determine, through the study of their chromosomes, if some of these tortoises had actually evolved into separate new species because of differing conditions on the islands—or if their chromosome counts were similar enough to show they remained subspecies of the Galápagos tortoise.

We finally concluded after much study that our tortoises were, in fact, still subspecies. We also discovered that incubation temperature played a key role in determining the sex of the hatchlings. In their natural habitat, tortoises and turtles lay their eggs on the beach or in sheltered areas on land that can be warm and sunny or cooler, depending on how much shade the nesting area gets. It turned out that the temperature of the incubating eggs established the hatchlings' sex. For years at the Zoo, we had been putting our tortoise and turtle eggs in an incubator and heating them at the same moderate temperature. The result was that all the babies were hatching as males! Up to this point, we had no way of realizing we were inadvertently causing this. Through our genetic chromosome analysis, we discovered that tortoises that incubated in warmer temperatures and in nests that are less shaded and more exposed to direct sun in the wild were more likely to hatch as females. We then changed the way we did things at the Zoo, and we wrote about it—as Dad insisted. Our research was starting to make a difference in areas no one had initially imagined.

Ollie discovered other firsts. Because of Dad's previous work with mules, donkeys, horses, and zebras, he called Ollie into his office one day and encouraged him to dive further into the study of the Przewalski's horse and other wild equids. Nobody had done a detailed study looking at the number of chromosomes and genetic structure. Ollie successfully applied for a three-year grant from the National Institutes of Health. The grant, which was renewed multiple times, ultimately led to 12 years of funding, enabling Ollie to purchase an ultracentrifuge and hire several technicians. He began exploring chromosomes in wild equids and how they might have evolved. It was fascinating . . . and good science. Along with a steady flow of publications in prestigious journals, the center's work continued to help raise the profile of the Zoo's wildlife research efforts.

This work studying the chromosomes of animals led to a new understanding of the different wildlife at the Zoo. It also led to greater reproductive success. One example was the Kirk's dik-dik, a beautiful and small ungulate (hoofed mammal) that most zoos, including the San Diego Zoo, just couldn't seem to breed. Some of the Zoos' original dik-diks that came from the wild produced offspring, but the offspring were always infertile and no one knew why. The problem, it turned out, was that zoos were importing animals that looked like Kirk's dik-diks but were, in fact, different species of dik-dik. Much like the famously infertile mule, the difference in chromosome counts among the imported hybrids was preventing successful breeding. This principle was the same for other species where reproduction efforts had failed. The research team's studies suddenly offered new hope for those efforts.

One addition to the staff around this time was Don Lindburg, an animal behaviorist from UCLA. He had a particular interest in lemurs, primates found only on the island of Madagascar. Their habitat was being destroyed at an alarming rate. Don soon established a breeding colony of ruffed lemurs at the Zoo to try to understand them further.

Another new staff member was Barbara Durrant, a postdoctoral researcher who had earned her PhD in reproductive physiology at North Carolina State University. When Dad hired Barbara, he made a point of asking her to report early for work on her first day. Wanting to make a good impression, Barbara arrived at the Scripps building—where she was told to go—at 7:30 in the morning, only to find the doors locked. She noticed a doorbell and pushed the button.

No one answered.

Barbara rang the bell again. Still no response. Wondering if she had missed something or was at the wrong building, she peeked through a window and saw a man wearing a bathrobe and slippers walking down the grand staircase. The man spotted Barbara and yelled from inside, "Who are you?"

Barbara panicked. Who was this half-dressed man? Clearly, she was in the wrong place. Now she was worried about being late on her first day, since she apparently still had to figure out where she was supposed to be!

But Barbara was in the right place after all. The man in the bathrobe turned out to be Bill Lasley, who was temporarily living in a small apartment on the second floor. Dad had forgotten to tell Bill, or anyone, that Barbara was coming. Dad also thought Barbara wasn't due to come in until the next day. Despite this mix-up and rocky beginning, Barbara returned the following morning to begin work that has lasted for more than 40 years (and counting).

Barbara's initial work was supposed to involve performing embryo transfers between different species of armadillos so the team could study multiple identical offspring. When she wasn't able to recover sufficient embryos for the project, she discovered through hormone analysis that the armadillos had progesterone levels that were abnormally high. This prevented them from reproducing. Barbara's study was over before it started. Her focus would shift to a new area, breeding endangered species—an effort that would take on increasing importance for the Zoo and for conservation efforts worldwide.

In November 1979, Dad hosted the World Conference on Breeding Endangered Species on behalf of the San Diego Zoo, an event that attracted more than 350 scientists from around the world. The conference was so successful that it spawned follow-up mini conferences that focused on problems around particular species. It was, Dad wrote, "a spectacular event. The city of San Diego, its Zoo, and the Wild Animal Park shone, and everything went just perfectly. All of us who were there will remember Roger Short's final speech, in which he held a gorilla skull high into the air, pleading for conservation of this unique species."

As the 1970s drew to a close, my father looked back with great pride on the previous five years and the achievements of his conservation research team. The important progress and impact they had made was clearly evident—enough so that the board of trustees granted more funds for another five years. Animal conservation and reproduction were becoming increasingly important for zoos and wildlife parks around the globe . . . and the San Diego Zoo was leading the way.

CHAPTER 16

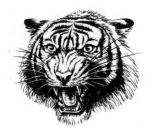

A Frozen Zoo

I n the fall of 1972, when I was still in high school, Dad and I made an exciting and unexpected discovery. The lagoons near San Diego lay along a north-south flyway traveled by migratory birds that we rarely saw otherwise. When the birds started heading south, I often brought Dad along for some early morning bird-watching. One foggy Saturday, we got up at 6 a.m. and drove north in my Volkswagen Bug along the coast highway that runs parallel to the beach. I spotted it first—a large, dark mass on the sand near the shallow water.

"What's that?" I asked, pointing to the lump on the beach.

Dad glanced over. "I don't know, but it looks interesting. Let's find out." We pulled over, climbed the sand dune separating the beach from the road, and walked down the deserted beach to the unusual object. It was a large, dead marine animal that must have washed up during the night. Almost 12 feet long, it was dark blue-gray along its back and pinkish on its belly. With a relatively large head and smaller lower jaw, it looked a little like a shark, but its body resembled a small whale.

"It's a whale," Dad said with excitement and conviction, "though I'm not sure what kind. Let's call Ulfur."

Ulfur Arneson, a Swedish scientist and friend who was an expert on whales, just happened to be in San Diego that week for a conference. After hearing our description, Ulfur said that we were probably looking at a pygmy sperm whale, a rare sighting. Dad and I took some pictures and then headed to the lagoon on the other side of the road to do our bird-watching. When we got home, we checked in with Ulfur, who had decided he really wanted to see the whale, so we picked him up at his hotel and returned to the beach.

Ulfur confirmed that the animal was indeed a pygmy sperm whale. He explained that since they were rarely seen in their native habitat, most of what we knew about them came from studying individuals that had washed up on beaches. Naturally, my father wanted a biopsy of the whale to add to his steadily expanding collection of animal tissue samples housed at the Frozen Zoo® (now part of the Wildlife Biodiversity Bank). He also wanted to count its chromosomes.

"I know you have a fascinating collection of skulls at your house," Ulfur mentioned as he and Dad were taking samples. "What do you think about adding a whale skull? You could take this one!"

"This skull is way too big," Dad said, shaking his head. "But maybe we could manage the lower jaw."

A moment later, Dad rolled up the sleeves of his ever-present dress shirt and went to work, sawing with a large knife until his arms were covered with the whale's blood. As the sun burned off the fog, a crowd of about 20 joggers and walkers gathered around us to watch. The two scientists succeeded in separating the jawbone from the rest of the carcass, and we put it into a plastic trash bag and transported it back to our home—much to Mom's consternation. She rolled her eyes when Dad carried our latest discovery into the kitchen, trailed by Ulfur. "Not another one!" she said. "Ulfur, if you weren't here, this is where I would draw the line."

"Oh, Marion," Dad teased, "you know you love doing this."

The jawbone was so big that we had to borrow a huge copper kettle from a friend so we could boil it clean, a procedure that took days. Mom had to figure out how to cook with this new science project in her kitchen, but when the process was over, we ended up with a beautiful white lower-jaw specimen to add to our collection. For the next several years, every time someone asked about or admired the jawbone, Mom would tell the tale of the pygmy sperm whale, rolling her eyes in mock disgust.

When I left to go bird-watching with Dad that day, I hadn't expected that we would spend most of our morning with a pygmy sperm whale. Yet it was in many ways a typical outing with my dad. You never knew what you might come across, and he was always ready to add to his collection of samples. One of his favorite quotes was by American historian Daniel Boorstin, who said, "You must collect things for reasons you don't yet understand." Dad considered his tissue samples an invaluable resource for study at the time, but he also felt that he was collecting for the future—even if he didn't exactly know how or why his specimens would be useful. He believed that the survival of tomorrow's endangered wildlife depended on the efforts made today.

When we first moved to San Diego, Dad flew back to New Hampshire to retrieve his collection, which was mostly made up of frozen samples. He bought a separate seat for the portable liquid nitrogen tank that held the samples and sat next to it on the flight back. Initially, he kept the samples in his lab at the university, but the Zoo eventually gave his collection a home in a room on the second floor of the newly formed research center. The frozen cells were transferred to what was basically a sophisticated freezer chest. The chest was roughly three feet square and filled with small glass vials (later switched to plastic). The samples were protected by glycerol and chilled in liquid nitrogen at minus 320 degrees Fahrenheit. The collection contained cell samples from hundreds of animals, including many that were near extinction: whales, antelope, rare cats, a giant armadillo, a greater one-horned rhinoceros, and a muntjac, to name just a few. Zoo officials began to recognize the significance of what Dad was doing. He ordered a plaque for the tissue bank that read, "The Frozen Zoo: 20th Century Ark."

At a news conference at the Zoo on July 25, 1974, my father and other Zoo officials talked about the importance of the cell bank. "Now is the time to collect," he said emphatically, "in order to protect future generations of animals." To emphasize the importance of taking immediate action, Dad revealed that the next day he was flying a sample of frozen sperm from the bonobo Kakowet—the Zoo's only male bonobo and one of fewer than 10 males in zoos—to New York and then to Belgium. The planned recipients of the sperm were three female bonobos at the Antwerp Zoo that would be impregnated via artificial insemination. (Bonobos, a great ape species, were extremely endangered and remain so today.)

Dad had seen the potential for saving wildlife through cell samples long before almost anyone else, and he now had the opportunity to do something about it. "It's not inconceivable," he said at the news conference, "to think that in the future, with these cell samples and the genetic code they carry, scientists with improved techniques available to them could accomplish the reconstruction of an animal that became extinct in our lifetime."

Sheldon Campbell, one of the Zoo trustees at the time, echoed Dad's comments, using the name my father had come up with for the collection of living cells. "This is the first cell bank started by any zoo, so far as we know," Campbell said. "The concept has all kinds of exciting possibilities, but perhaps the most intriguing is the idea of creating a 'frozen zoo' today which might someday enable us to reproduce species which have become extinct."

Collecting and preserving fragile, living material in hopes that it may one day lead to renewed life for a species is not an easy business. In 1977, the guardians of the Frozen Zoo were reminded just how precarious that effort could be. Though her title was never official, Arlene Kumamoto took over the daily responsibility of serving as curator of the Frozen Zoo. At the time, its liquid nitrogen tank included an alarm to warn staff members if anything went wrong, but the alarm was so quiet that it could be heard only from inside the room where it was located. One morning, Arlene arrived for work and discovered a failure in the nitrogen tank. The tank's precious contents were thawing.

Horrified, Arlene enlisted the help of staff member Mark Bogart. Together, they spent the next 24 hours emptying the contents of each vial into tissue culture flasks, which they placed in an incubator in hopes of reviving the cells. Sadly, it was too late. The entire collection was lost—more than 350 tissue samples, most of them already grown into cell lines, representing years of Dad's patient work. Among the most significant losses were cell lines from a blue whale and a northern white rhino, both highly endangered. Other material that was difficult to replace, because the animals could no longer be found in North American zoos, included samples from a fairy armadillo, giant armadillo, green acouchi, Chinese ferret badger, olingo, masked civet, and fur seal. The sample from our pygmy sperm whale was also lost.

Dad and the staff were devastated. But my father wasn't one to dwell on setbacks. "Okay," he said in his matter-of-fact way, "let's just start over again." He and the staff installed a better alarm system, and a new technician was hired to help rebuild the collection of samples. Dad added a second nitrogen tank to serve as a backup, housing duplicates of the material kept in the first tank.

His worries were not over, however. On the evening of March 8, 1978, an arsonist struck at the historic Old Globe theatre in San Diego's Balboa Park, igniting a three-alarm fire that razed the theater and sent bright orange flames high into the night sky. The back of the theater was across from the front door of the offices in the Scripps building, with only a narrow street separating the two. Arlene, who lived nearby, saw the smoke and hurried over to check on the situation, watching as firefighters battled to keep the fire from spreading to the Zoo and elsewhere.

Everyone was relieved that the fire didn't extend to the Scripps building or the Zoo, but Dad knew it was a narrow escape. The incident seemed to be symbolic of the uncertain future for wildlife and how important it was to preserve and expand this work.

Dad and the researchers were gradually increasing the collection of cell samples when Barbara Durrant began her postdoctoral work at the Zoo in 1979. Though her initial attempts to study armadillo reproduction had been thwarted, she still had grant money available to fulfill her postdoctoral study. She needed a new project. Dad suggested she work with Bill Lasley, who invited Barbara to do hormone assays in the endocrine lab. Barbara, however, had another idea. Through the window of her lab on the first floor of the Scripps building, she had a view of the room used for the Zoo's animal necropsies.

"When the doors were open," she remembers, "I could see what the veterinarians were doing in there. I watched them take sections but then discard the rest of the carcass, and I thought, 'That's a lot of sperm and eggs we could be using for study.'"

First, however, Barbara had to convince my dad. She knew how busy he was, so she was nervous about interrupting his schedule to propose a shift in his plan for her research. When she approached him, he was dressed in his usual shirt and tie, his head buried in his work.

"There are already several people in the endocrine lab doing assays," Barbara began. "I don't feel that I would be adding much value if that was all I did. But I've been seeing a rich resource of sperm and eggs coming through necropsy every day and have an idea."

Dad was still looking down at his paperwork, but he was listening. Barbara explained that she hoped to explore how to cryopreserve not just cell samples of animals but reproductive material to advance research and conservation. The Frozen Zoo had no reproductive samples in its collection at the time. In fact, in the late 1970s, only domestic livestock sperm were being frozen anywhere, so protocols were scarce. "I don't know much about sperm," Barbara said, talking in a rush, "but I know a lot about eggs and embryos. I can learn what I don't know."

Dad finally looked up and made eye contact. "You've sold me," he said. "That's a good idea. Go do it." With that simple confirmation, the future for Barbara Durrant and the Frozen Zoo changed dramatically.

Developing protocols for freezing reproductive material required extensive research, as every animal species was different. In March 1980, Barbara successfully banked semen from an addax (an antelope) in the liquid nitrogen tank. It was the beginning of the Zoo's Germplasm Repository, which included reproductive material saved for future research, breeding, and conservation. Soon after, she banked material from a Grevy's zebra—the first ovarian tissue in the Frozen Zoo.

Around this time, Dad had another conversation with Barbara. "It is very clear that we need to continue collecting sperm and eggs and preserve them," he said. "This will be important in the future. How would you like to work here permanently?"

"I would love that," she replied with a huge smile. The opportunity to apply her skills and education to the conservation of endangered wildlife was everything she could ask for in a career.

"He took a chance on me as a postdoc," Barbara recalls today. "Then he took a chance on me as an employee in offering me a full-time job. I owe my entire career to Dr. B."

Dad subsequently approved a formal new reproductive physiology division. That early study of freezing gametes (cells that can join together to create life) put the San Diego Zoo at the forefront of the effort to freeze reproductive materials and helped launch the field of exotic animal cryopreservation research. It also helped define Barbara's work for the next 40-plus years. As of 2022, she is the Henshaw Endowed Director of Reproductive Sciences for San Diego Zoo Wildlife Alliance. She and her staff study reproductive biology, endocrinology, and behavior, and they continue to develop innovative methods to further reproduction.

"The importance of this work cannot be overemphasized," Barbara says. "Saving these resources will allow us, and those who follow, to genetically reinvigorate populations and mitigate some of the effects of population declines. When the Frozen Zoo was conceived, no one knew how the cells might be used in the future, but Dr. B knew they *must* be saved or be lost forever. He saw the need when few others did."

It was indeed a "good idea"—one that is still making a difference for endangered wildlife today.

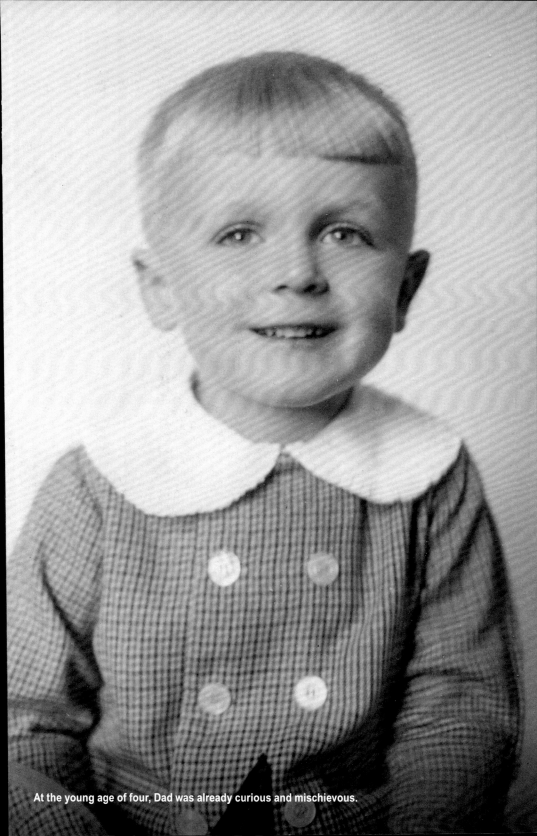
At the young age of four, Dad was already curious and mischievous.

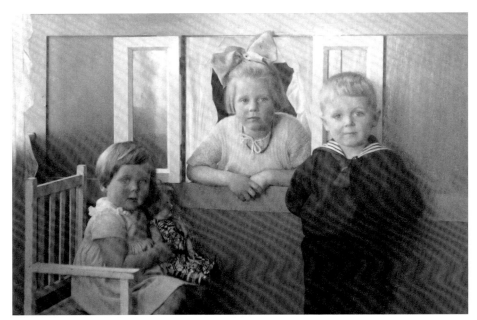
Dad loved his sisters Lotte (left) and Ilse (center) but was less fond of their playhouse.

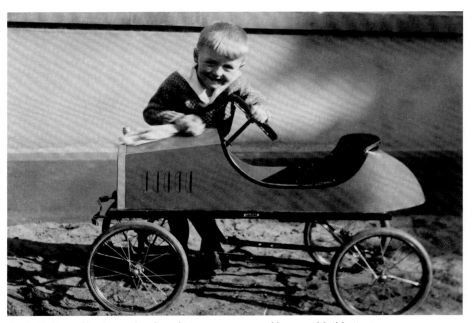
My dad's love of fast cars developed at a young age and began with this toy car.

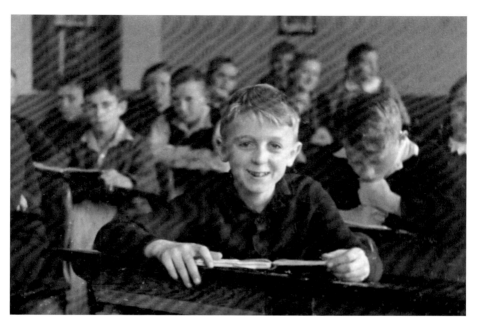
While he was very bright, Dad was not always the most dedicated student, so his teachers often seated him at the front of the class.

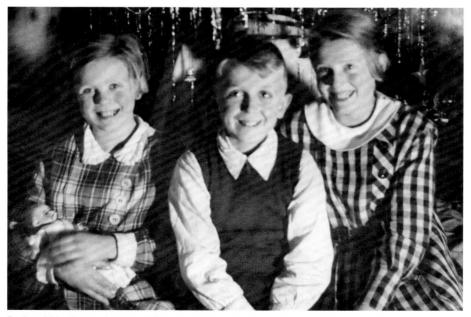
Dad and his sisters, Lotte and Ilse, dressed up for the holidays in Glückstadt, Germany.

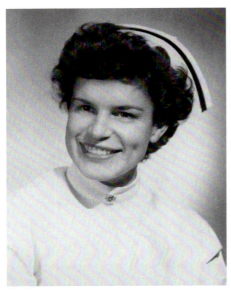
Marion Waldhausen—my mom—was the bright and beautiful young nurse who won Dad's heart.

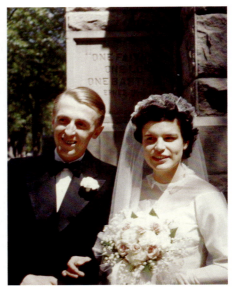
Dad and Mom were married on May 17, 1952, in Great Falls, Montana.

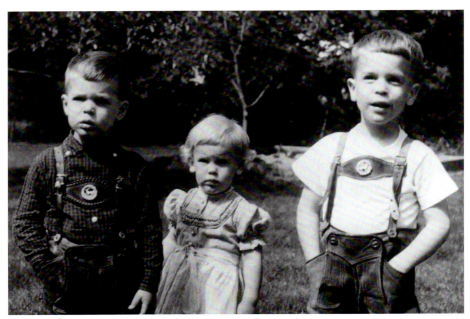
Our parents frequently dressed us in traditional German attire: lederhosen (leather pants) for me (left) and Steve and a dirndl for Ingrid.

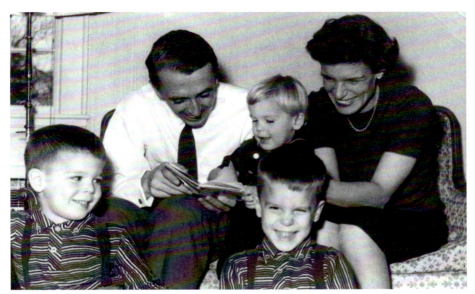

Each year, our family sent out a Christmas card featuring a family photo that Dad took, developed, and printed in his own darkroom. This photo is from 1958.

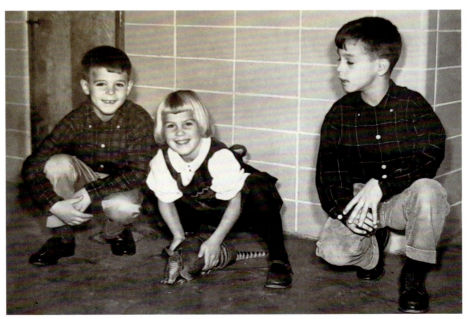

Ingrid, Steve, and I had fun spending time with an armadillo in Dad's lab at Dartmouth's medical school in the early 1960s.

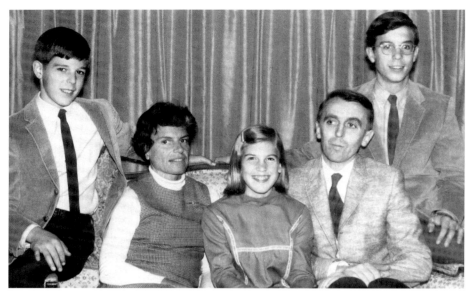

Our last Christmas in Hanover, New Hampshire, was in 1969. We moved to California the following year.

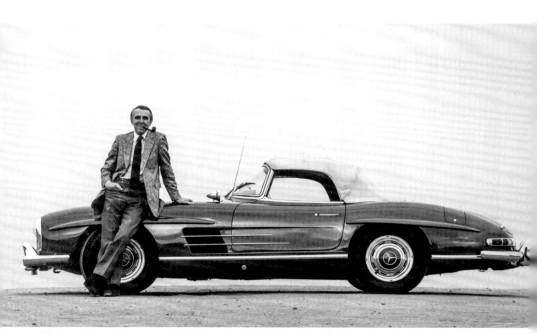

Dad's pride and joy was a 1960 Mercedes 300 SL Roadster that he and my brother, Steve, restored together.

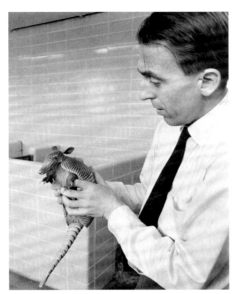

Dad was fascinated to discover that armadillos produced quadruplets every time they had offspring.

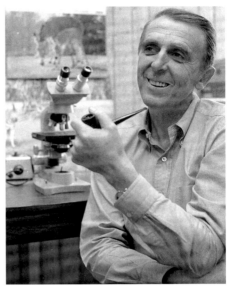

My dad—pictured in his office at the San Diego Zoo—was most relaxed when spending time in the lab.

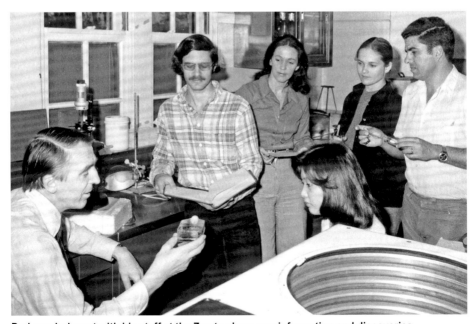

Dad regularly met with his staff at the Zoo to share new information and discoveries.

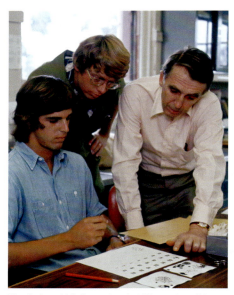

My dad and bird curator Art Risser taught me a lot about bird chromosomes during one of my summer internships at the San Diego Zoo.

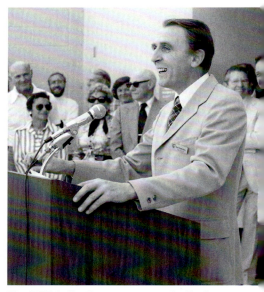

The 1977 dedication ceremony at the Zoo's new veterinary hospital featured Dad as one of the speakers.

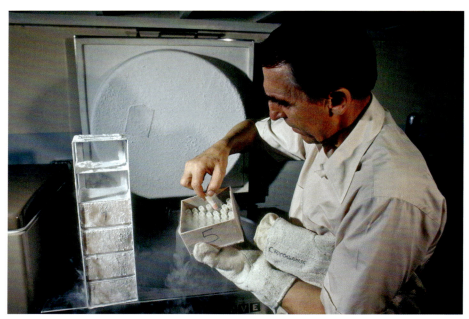

Dad's creation of the Frozen Zoo continues to impact the preservation of endangered species today.

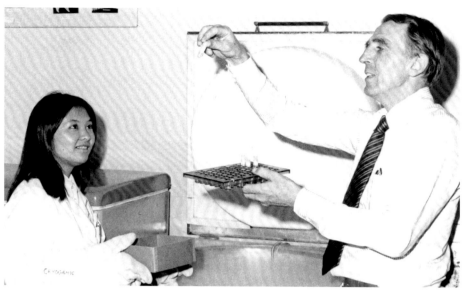

Arlene Kumamoto, who became an international authority on animal cytogenetics, was one of my dad's favorite colleagues.

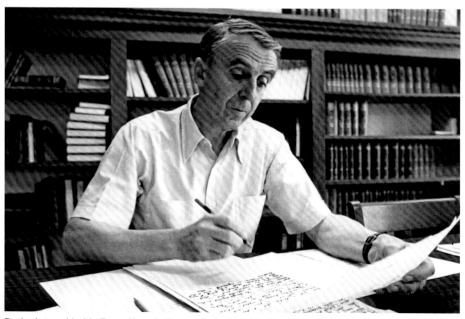

Dad, pictured in his Zoo office, believed strongly in the importance of writing and publishing his findings in scientific journals to share knowledge and advance the field.

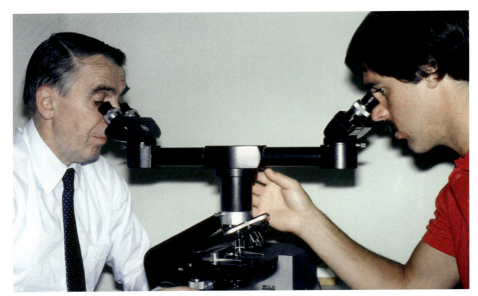

When I wasn't playing football for the San Diego Chargers, I often spent time in the Zoo's lab with my father, learning about chromosomes.

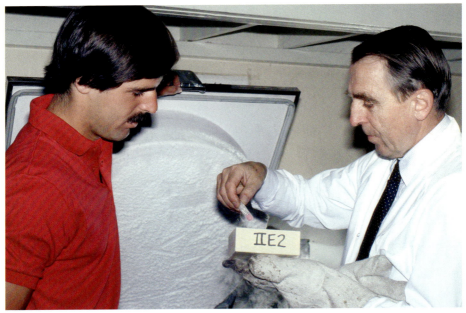

Dad liked to show me samples from the Frozen Zoo and explain new breakthroughs that were happening.

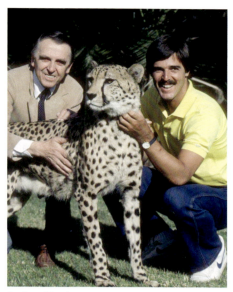

Dad and I enjoyed a moment with Arusha the cheetah, one of the Zoo's wildlife ambassadors, in 1983.

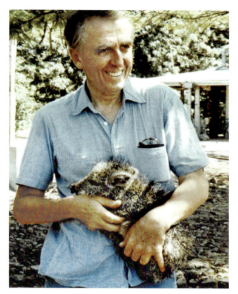

Dad, holding a Chacoan peccary in Paraguay, was instrumental in saving this rare species from extinction.

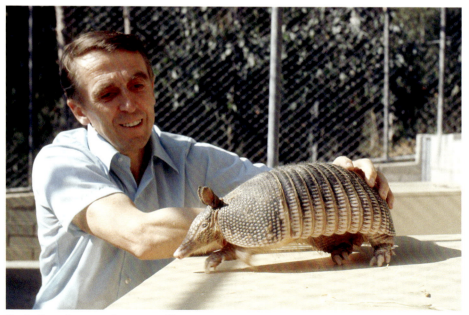

My dad's early research on armadillos at Dartmouth continued at the San Diego Zoo.

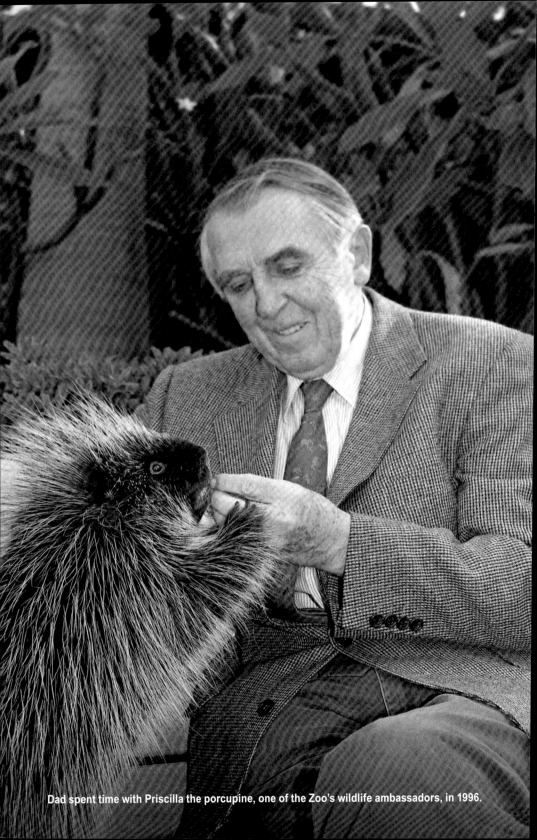
Dad spent time with Priscilla the porcupine, one of the Zoo's wildlife ambassadors, in 1996.

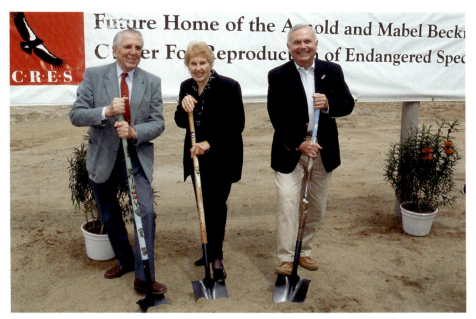
Patricia Beckman and Zoo trustee Bill May helped Dad break ground in 2003 for the new conservation headquarters funded by Patricia's parents, Arnold and Mabel Beckman.

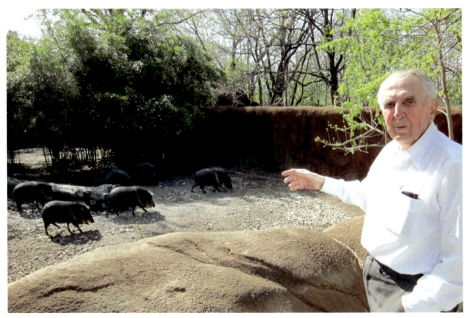
With the support of the International Union for Conservation of Nature (IUCN), my father cocreated a Species Survival Plan for the rare Chacoan peccary.

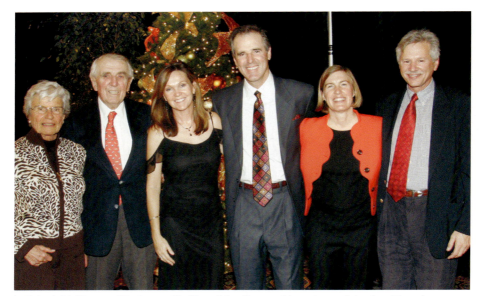

Left to right: Mom and Dad; my wife, Mary (standing next to me); my sister, Ingrid; and her husband, Gordon, celebrated with me when I received the San Diego Zoo's esteemed Conservation Medal in December 2007.

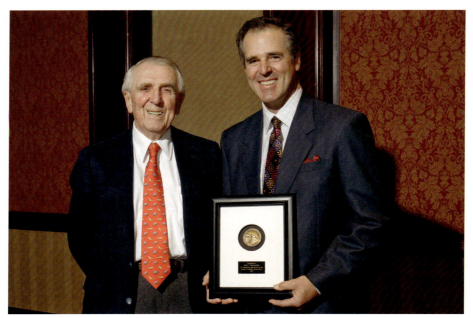

I was honored to celebrate with my father, whose own passion for science, conservation, and wildlife inspired me from an early age.

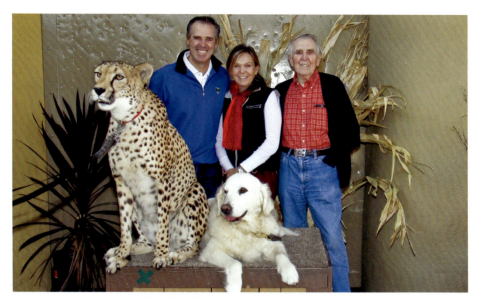

During a visit to the Zoo in 2011, Dad, Mary, and I spent time with Karroo the cheetah and her companion, Sven Olaf the golden retriever.

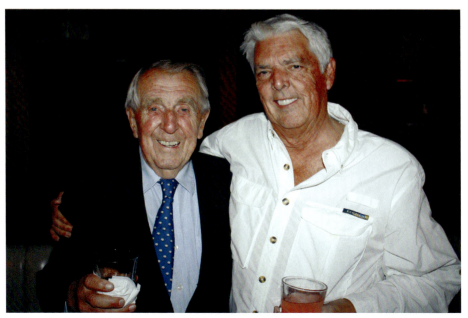

Dr. Dave Fagan, a wildlife dental specialist, was one of Dad's dearest friends for four decades.

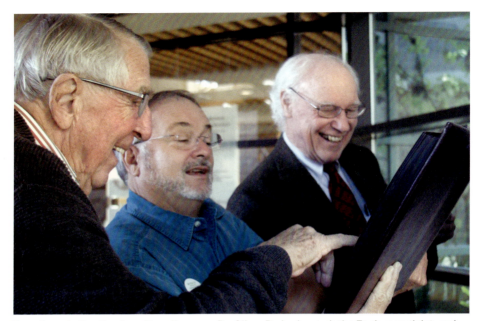

Two of my dad's other favorite colleagues, Dr. Oliver Ryder (center), the Zoo's geneticist, and Dr. Ken Jones from UCSD, reminisced with him about a project they had worked on together.

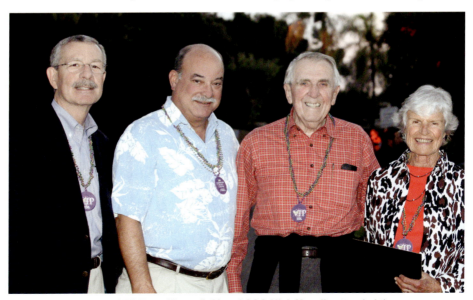

The Zoo's now-retired CEO Doug Myers (left) and COO Mick Musella attended the Celebration for the Critters with Mom and Dad in 2009. Now called the San Diego Zoo Food, Wine & Brew Celebration, the event continues to raise funds for wildlife conservation.

CHAPTER 17

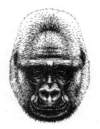

ONE MEDICINE

Our relationship with the environment has enormous implications for human health. This idea can be traced back at least as far as the 5th century BC and the writings of the Greek physician Hippocrates. In the mid-1800s, German physician Rudolf Virchow, known as the father of modern pathology, recognized a similar link between animal and human medicine. He advocated for veterinary medical education and came up with the term "zoonosis" to describe a disease that can be passed from animals to humans. Yet by the 20th century, few seemed ready to acknowledge the commonalities between human and animal physiology and the potential benefits of studying and applying them together. Instead, human and veterinary medicine evolved into separate disciplines.

One of the first people to propose merging these disciplines was Dr. Calvin Schwabe, a founding faculty member of the UC Davis School of Medicine and an epidemiology professor at the UC Davis School of Veterinary Medicine.

Dr. Schwabe has been credited with coining the term "One Medicine" in a book published in 1964 to describe this approach. Dr. Schwabe served with my father on the National Research Council, and they became good friends.

Like Dr. Schwabe, Dad was able to see what others did not. Ever since he had done comparative twinning research on armadillos back in the 1950s, Dad had recognized that the things we learn about animals can be applied to the human body and human health, and vice versa. He became more convinced of this during his visits to the Catskill Game Park and as he expanded his study of animal chromosomes. It made little sense, Dad reasoned, to differentiate between human and veterinary medicine. Why not combine knowledge and medical practices for all species? As he wrote in 1987, "I strongly believe in the 'One Medicine' concept, that few essential differences exist in the diagnosis and therapy of most human diseases and those of animals. Thus, a confluence of these disciplines is highly desirable."

In the late 1970s, during his conversations with Bill Lasley at the two-headed microscope, Dad discussed his hope that One Medicine could achieve equity, harmony, and collaboration among medical professionals and veterinarians. He put that idea into practice, frequently asking the Zoo veterinary staff for advice or permission to explore his latest theory. Although some members of the veterinary staff were initially resistant to the idea of a medical doctor infringing on their domain, Dad gradually won them over. He nearly always supported the veterinarians' decisions and activities, and they developed a collaborative partnership.

Around the time that the conservation research department was formed, my dad met David Fagan, a dentist who had just moved to San Diego and would become one of Dad's closest colleagues and friends. Dave had considerable experience with both human and veterinary dentistry, including large-animal surgery at the UC Davis Veterinary Medical Teaching Hospital. Colleagues in Davis had urged Dave to contact Dad. "Find Benirschke," one of them said. "You'll enjoy him."

Dave visited Dad at his office, sharing about his passion for veterinary dentistry. Dad was quick to recognize the possibilities for One Medicine that Dave presented. "What are you doing today?" Dad asked. "Nothing? Come with me. Let's see if we've got any problems."

He immediately took Dave to meet Phil Robinson, DVM, the Zoo's director of veterinary services. That led to a meeting with Jim Oosterhuis, DVM, director of veterinary services for the Wild Animal Park. In no time, Dave found himself serving as the staff dentistry consultant for both the Zoo and the Park. With continued encouragement from Dad, Dave began working closely with Phil Robinson and Jim Oosterhuis. They developed a program to methodically examine the dental needs of the animals at the Zoo and Park—roughly 3,000 mammals.

In Dave Fagan, my father had found a kindred spirit, particularly in relation to the practice of medicine among different species. Dave later wrote, "Essentially there are only minor differences between a surgical procedure in the mouth of a human, called human dentistry; a surgical procedure in the abdomen of a child, called human medicine; and a surgical procedure on the leg of a monkey, called veterinary medicine. With relatively minor—albeit critical and sophisticated—variations, the practice of all three of these different medicines is essentially just different forms of the practice of mammalian medicine. When it is all said and done, we are after all just a bunch of mammals. The clinical reality of all this is that there is just *one medicine*."

For Dave, a thorough review of dental issues at the Zoo and Park was only the beginning. Shortly after the 1977 opening of the Zoo's new veterinary hospital, Phil Robinson called on Dave to perform the hospital's first clinical procedure. Akabori, a female leopard native to North China, underwent a successful dental surgery to repair external root reabsorption and multiple abscesses, which were the result of an unusually destructive form of periodontal disease.

In 1978, Dave performed his first examination of a gorilla. Trib, a 19-year-old lowland silverback, was the dominant male gorilla at the Wild Animal Park. He stood taller than 6 feet and weighed 432 pounds. But Trib had stopped eating and was listless and dull-eyed—and no one could figure out why. When Dave peered into the gorilla's mouth, four times the size of an adult human's mouth, he found cauliflower-shaped growths with magenta-colored margins. He also smelled the foul odor of dying gingival tissue. Trib's entire mouth was acutely inflamed and badly infected.

Dave's experience with human patients gave him the clues to solve the problem. Because he had read Trib's medical history, he knew that Trib suffered from seizures and had recently begun taking medication. He also knew that humans taking a certain medication for epilepsy could develop ulcerative gingivitis. Though the connection had never been reported in veterinary literature, Dave believed that the medication's effect would be the same for a gorilla.

Thanks to this insight, the Zoo reduced Trib's medication dosage and put the gorilla on antibiotics. Dave then treated Trib with a full mouth gingivectomy and removed his impacted molars. Trib regained his health and continued to be the patriarch of the Park's lowland gorilla troop for another 15 years.

Of all the animals Dave treated at the Zoo and Park, Trib was one of his favorites. The big silverback exuded a majesty and dignity as well as a sense of compassion. Dave liked to tell the story of a wildlife care specialist who accidentally hit her finger with a hammer while hanging up a calendar. When Trib heard her cry out in pain, he came over to investigate on his side of the habitat. The specialist held out her hand for him to see. Unexpectedly, Trib slowly extended one finger through the barrier and gently stroked her injury. The specialist later told Dave that the tenderness she felt from Trib at that moment surpassed anything she'd experienced from another human. When Trib died in 1993 from a ruptured aortic aneurysm, Dave and many others felt as if they'd lost a close friend.

Years earlier, Dave had shared with Dad how difficult it was for him when an animal died after intense efforts to keep it healthy. "Failure is a constant companion in the zoo world," Dad commiserated. "Clearly, we're going to lose from time to time. The practice of medicine is, to a great extent, a never-ending battle. You won't win the war—there are just too many diseases—but you can win skirmishes and be thankful for that."

Dave's work over the years included creating a prosthetic to repair the shattered beak of an eagle, grafting bone into the jawbones of a Malayan tiger, and removing an enormous partial tooth that had merged with a normal molar in the mouth of a female Asian elephant. The latter, which involved the use of a six-foot steel crowbar, was the most difficult and physically demanding surgical procedure Dave ever performed.

When Dave started his work with the Zoo, dentistry as a functional discipline of veterinary medicine was virtually nonexistent. He had to create techniques and protocols as he went along. With help from Dad and Phil Robinson, Dave designed and built a mobile dental unit that with minor modifications could provide complete dental care for any animal, anywhere around the country, at any time. Dad also encouraged Dave to publish his work. "Kurt pushed me constantly," says Dave. "I remember early on he told me, 'You know, Fagan, you have a paucity of publications! You should work on correcting that!' So I worked harder." Dave went on to publish more than 40 papers that described his many discoveries and insights in detail, and he significantly advanced the emerging field of zoo dentistry.

Dad also impressed upon Dave the need for an entity that would facilitate further study of oral-related medical issues in animals and create awareness of the need for veterinary dental knowledge. In 1982, with Dad's help as one of the founding directors, Dave established the Colyer Institute, a nonprofit organization that conducts clinical dental care in facilities around the globe, performs research, and establishes education programs for related veterinary, wildlife, and public communities. The institute has embraced my father's message about the importance of mentorship, preparing a second generation of staff to continue its work.

In reflecting on his long career in veterinary dentistry and the changes in veterinary medicine, Dave says that Dad's impact can't be overstated. "Kurt Benirschke is to the zoo world what Winston Churchill is to international politics," Dave says unabashedly. "He's had a huge, huge influence all around the globe."

∞

Dentistry was just one example of how Dad sought to connect human medicine and the veterinary community. Robert "Bob" Resnik remembers the day in 1977 that my dad came into his office at UCSD. A female douc langur at the Zoo—a critically endangered primate native to Southeast Asia—was carrying a fetus that had died but hadn't yet been delivered, and the staff had serious concerns for the mother's health.

"Would you come down," Dad asked Bob, "and do a Caesarean section on her?"

Bob—a UCSD faculty member and perinatologist who later directed the university's department of obstetrics, gynecology, and reproductive sciences—briefly pondered the question. He had performed numerous C-sections on women, but never on an animal, let alone an endangered one. Bob knew, of course, that the physiology between humans and primates was similar, and he reasoned that this was an opportunity to help an animal in distress and perhaps learn something at the same time. Besides, who could say "no" to Kurt Benirschke?

As Dad and Bob discussed the upcoming procedure, they decided to take blood samples from the douc langur to test for any potential abnormalities. On the day of the surgery at the Zoo hospital, Dad scrubbed in and assisted Bob and the Zoo's veterinary team. The procedure was a success and saved the mother from further complications. More interesting, however, was that the blood tests revealed a clotting abnormality that indicated dead fetus syndrome. This condition likely would have led the mother to experience massive bleeding had she delivered the fetus naturally. It was the first time that anyone had observed dead fetus syndrome in a nonhuman. My father and Bob were ecstatic that their intuition to proceed with the operation had saved such a rare animal. Naturally, they published a paper about it.

In 1981, Dad was back in Bob's office with another problem. "We've got a pregnant lowland gorilla at the Wild Animal Park," he explained. "We're all concerned about the fetus because during the gorilla's previous pregnancy, the fetus died. What do you think we should do?"

"Why don't we do an amniocentesis and see if the lungs are mature?" Bob suggested. "If they're developed enough, I'll do a Cesarean section." As far as they knew, no one had ever performed an amniocentesis or a C-section on a gorilla, but that didn't deter them.

At 5 a.m. on April 23, 1981, a team of specialists from UCSD's medical faculty—including Louis Gluck, founder of the world's first neonatal intensive care unit and developer of the procedure for determining fetal lung maturity—arrived at the Wild Animal Park to meet Dad and the Park staff. The sun was just peeking over the hills of San Pasqual Valley when a veterinarian approached the habitat of the prospective gorilla parents—Dolly, the pregnant mother, due in two months, and Trib, the father.

The vet shot a dart at Dolly to sedate her. When the medication took hold and she lay down, her uncomprehending partner was not happy. Trib pounded his chest and roared at the humans. George Leopold, who was in charge of the ultrasound that day, calmly winked at Trib, pointed at Bob, and said, "It was Resnik who did it!"

The wildlife care specialists were able to call Trib to a separate area, and the team moved the sedated Dolly. They performed an ultrasound that clearly showed that the baby gorilla inside Dolly was healthy but that the baby's lungs weren't yet mature enough for a birth. After much discussion, Bob and the team decided to hold off on doing a C-section and instead monitor the situation closely. Their caution paid off. Two months later, Dolly delivered a healthy baby gorilla that was named Mary Ellen.

With Dad's encouragement and leadership, cooperation and collaboration between UCSD's medical faculty and the Zoo's research and veterinary staffs continued to grow. Experts in human and veterinary medicine combined their knowledge and skills, and more procedures, new discoveries, and published papers occurred as a result. The concept of One Medicine was becoming a reality.

Perhaps the best example of One Medicine in action—and the procedure that required the greatest degree of planning and number of human volunteers—took place at the San Diego Zoo on August 27, 1994. During a veterinary exam earlier that year, a Zoo veterinarian discovered a heart murmur in Karen, a nearly two-year-old endangered Sumatran orangutan (today, the species is critically endangered). Dad found a cardiologist who normally treated humans and convinced him to perform an ultrasound on Karen. The procedure showed that Karen had an atrial septal defect (ASD), a hole in the wall between the two upper chambers of her heart. Untreated, the congenital defect could lead to irreversible lung damage.

ASD closure was a fairly common operation on human babies, but as far as anyone could determine, it had never been done on an orangutan. Two world-famous cardiac surgeons, Dr. Stuart Jamieson and Dr. Jolene Kriett, donated their time for the surgery. Planning for the operation was extensive. Dad and Dr. Kriett met for hours with a team of surgeons, anesthesiologists, nurses, blood bank specialists, veterinarians, and wildlife care specialists to coordinate the procedure. In all, more than 100 specialists participated in Karen's historic seven-hour surgery and her recovery.

The operation went well, although Karen developed complications that required the rapid creation of an intensive care unit and round-the-clock care for two weeks following the surgery. Ultimately, however, Karen made a full recovery and was returned to her habitat at the Zoo, where she continues to thrive today.

The intensive care unit became an established addition at the Zoo, and numerous other animals at the Zoo benefited from it over time. Once again, pioneering cooperation between experts in human and animal medicine led to new advances and greater understanding. As Don Janssen, DVM, retired corporate director of animal health at San Diego Zoo Global, put it, "One of the greatest benefits of this new cooperation was the educational interchange between two healing professions that really do have a lot in common."

For our father's 60th birthday on May 26, 1984, my mom, brother, and I joined Dad's colleagues and friends to celebrate both the man and his leadership in the One Medicine movement. (Work commitments kept Ingrid in New York.)

It was a surprise party, no easy feat to pull off. As we drove to the Wild Animal Park, Dad believed he was heading to a small family celebration. Instead, we walked up to the beautiful, grassy meadow with views of the Park's African Plains, where more than 50 colleagues and friends had gathered. Some of the guests had traveled from across the country and even halfway around the world, including Dennis Meritt, assistant director of Chicago's Lincoln Park Zoo; Lorna Johnson, pathologist at the New England Primate Research Center; and Hiroaki Soma from the Department of Obstetrics and Gynecology at Tokyo Medical College.

When Dad saw the crowd and grasped what was happening, a huge smile lit up his face. He shook his head in disbelief. Our father, who rarely showed much emotion despite feeling it deeply, was clearly touched by this demonstration of respect and love from his close friends and the people he admired most. For the first time in my life, I saw Dad uncomfortable and speechless, unable to put into words what this genuine expression of love and appreciation meant to him.

The event included remarks from Sheldon Campbell, then president of the Zoological Society of San Diego, and other guests, followed by a video presentation and slides portraying Dad's life. Steve, Mom, and I had the chance to say a few words to honor him, and the three of us kids also wrote a note that was in the program. It stated, "Although we don't know everyone personally, we have heard your names around the dinner table many times and know how special each of you is to Dad. You are his colleagues, coworkers, and friends, and are what make his life so interesting and rewarding. To you, he is a scientist, teacher, leader, and friend with whom you have shared many experiences. To us, he is our father, and we love him."

The party concluded with the special presentation of a *Festschrift*, a volume of writings from many different colleagues given in tribute to a respected academic leader. The tradition originated in Germany prior to World War I. Dad's *Festschrift* was a hardbound, limited-edition book made up of original papers written by colleagues and people who admired and were influenced by his work. Ollie Ryder and Mary (Byrd) Cole spearheaded the enormous effort to create it and asked many of Dad's colleagues from the Zoo and medical world as well as former students to contribute. The effort resulted in nearly 30 original scientific papers from 62 authors, including important figures in pathology, genetics, and veterinary medicine from San Diego and around the world. The simple title of the volume, printed by Springer-Verlag, his longtime publisher, said it best: *One Medicine: A Tribute to Kurt Benirschke*.

In the book's foreword, Springer-Verlag publisher Dr. Heinz Götze wrote about Dad's commitment and connection to nature: "He might be considered a modern adept of the Greek and Roman Stoic school of philosophy, which taught an understanding of man as integrated into nature in its totality. The right way to live is according to nature, with nature as part of it. This at the same time means humanity, and Kurt Benirschke impresses us not only as an outstanding scientist but also as a humanist who has had a lifelong love affair with nature." In the book's introduction, Ollie and Mary wrote, "We attempt to recognize the breadth and depth of his thinking and to acknowledge the significant role he played in aspects of human medicine, veterinary medicine, and wildlife conservation."

The book came with a separate stack of congratulatory letters from research associates and colleagues in San Diego and from around the world—experts in, fittingly, both human and animal medicine. Dad couldn't stop smiling and shaking his head in disbelief at what so many people had done to honor him. As I watched the sun begin to dip beneath the hills, painting the sky a picturesque crimson, I knew this was an evening he and all of us would never forget.

PART 5
WORLDWIDE

Advancing
Knowledge

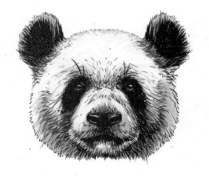

CHAPTER 18

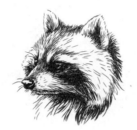

A Pain in the Gut

My father, Kurt Benirschke, was used to achieving whatever he put his mind to. He had overcome many obstacles in his life, including surviving a world war, learning a new language, adapting to a new country, and finding success in the complex arena of medicine. He became an expert in perinatal pathology and genetics, the world's foremost authority on the placenta, and a leading figure in the fields of veterinary medicine and conservation science. Yet as successful as Dad was, some things were beyond even his abilities. Unexpected events in my life would challenge us both—and ultimately lead to a dramatic change in our relationship.

It started on September 9, 1978, with stomach cramps that I figured were the result of the fast-food burger I'd eaten for lunch. At the time, I was just beginning my second season playing in the NFL for the San Diego Chargers, who'd claimed me from the Oakland Raiders the year before. I had successfully made the transition from college to the pros and had become a reliable kicker and an important contributor to our young team. The Chargers had not played very well during my rookie season, but we were hoping to improve.

But the pain in my abdomen that evening didn't go away. I started having diarrhea, increasing pain, and a low-grade fever. When my problems persisted, I finally told my parents, and Dad arranged for me to see a UCSD doctor and undergo a series of tests. I'll never forget the doctor's words after he called me in.

"Based on these X-rays and your fever, your tender abdomen, and your bloody diarrhea, you may have an inflammatory bowel disease known as Crohn's disease," he said without a hint of emotion.

"What the heck is Crohn's disease?" I asked anxiously.

"It's a chronic disease we don't know much about," he responded, "and at the moment there is no known cure."

No cure! I hardly heard anything else the doctor said. I was in shock. That night, Dad led me into his study, which was lined with dozens of medical books, and we started to read about Crohn's disease. We learned that it was one of two inflammatory bowel diseases (ulcerative colitis being the other) that typically affected the small intestine but could develop in any part of the digestive tract. The cause of the disease was unknown, and it affected patients in a range of ways. Sometimes it went into remission when patients took certain medications, but often patients required surgery—even multiple surgeries—to remove parts of their intestines. We also discovered that some patients needed an ostomy, where an opening would be surgically created in the abdomen for the intestine to divert bodily wastes into an ostomy pouch attached to the patient's side.

Dad was very concerned, and I was scared.

Over the next six weeks, my doctor tried to manage the inflammation, my abdominal pain, and my ongoing diarrhea with the drugs that were available at the time. I continued to try to kick for the Chargers, but I was losing weight and felt my strength ebbing. One night, after stopping over at my parents' house for dinner, I just couldn't keep my emotions bottled up anymore. I broke down and shared my frustrations and fears with them. Mom was very empathetic, but it was hard for Dad to hear. He had spent his entire life helping people and animals with his vast knowledge of science and medicine, but now he couldn't even help his own son. He wasn't a patient person anyway, and he finally reached the point where he just couldn't listen to me anymore.

"Quit bitching and fight harder," he snapped at me. "Take control of this. Maybe you should get out of this stupid football anyway. Get a real job. Then maybe you can get away from the stress of all this."

That hurt.

"Dad, this isn't caused by stress and football!" I said. "Everything we've read says it isn't, and you know that. If I stop playing football, what then? There's no guarantee this disease is going to go away, and then I'm just sick without a job! I'm fighting as best I can. I'm doing everything I can. Do you think I *like* being sick?"

A few minutes later, after Dad had left the room, Mom sat next to me and put her arm around my shoulders. "You know Dad didn't mean what he said," she told me gently. "He's just worried. He doesn't know how to handle this, and we both wish there was something we could do for you. You know how Dad is. He feels things so deeply, but he sometimes doesn't know how to express his emotions."

I knew she was right, but it was still pretty tough to hear my father say that I wasn't trying hard enough to get healthy or that being in the NFL wasn't a "real job." I managed to finish out the season with the Chargers, but my health was deteriorating. It got so bad that for the final few weeks of the season, I kicked on Sunday and then spent the remainder of the week in the hospital getting fed via an IV in my neck. I would check out of the hospital on Saturday afternoon, spend the night with the team at the hotel, play the game on Sunday, and get readmitted to the hospital Sunday night. It was crazy, but I didn't know what else to do.

That season, our team had brought in a new coach, Don Coryell, and our offense couldn't be stopped. We were getting good, and the city of San Diego had fallen in love with our team. I got a lot of chances to kick and wanted to keep playing if at all possible. I spent that offseason trying every treatment the doctors prescribed as well as a few that I had heard about from other Crohn's disease sufferers. I adjusted my diet, got a lot of rest, and trained as hard as my body allowed me to. The piercing cramps and diarrhea continued, but I convinced myself I was getting better.

I started my third season in 1979 with high hopes, and I was able to retain my job kicking for the Chargers. Then in the second week of the season, after kicking an extra point in a game against Oakland, I took a late hit that fractured three ribs and left me in severe pain. From there, my health and strength declined further, but with the help of pain-numbing injections for my ribs, I continued kicking. Two games later, we traveled to Boston to play the New England Patriots. We lost 27–21, our first defeat of the season. I didn't know it at the time, but it was the last game I would play that year.

On the team plane flying home after the game, I collapsed in the aisle with a 103-degree fever. The next morning, I was taken to the doctor, and after further tests, the decision I'd hoped to avoid was finally made: I needed surgery, and my season was finished. I was devastated. I didn't have much time to mourn, though. I was immediately checked into UCSD's University Hospital, and things continued to get more serious.

To make matters worse for our family, my sister, Ingrid, who was on her very first business trip, went to the emergency room in Minneapolis for severe side and back pain. She had kidney stones and needed surgery. Ingrid decided to have her operation in San Diego. Loaded up on painkillers, she flew from Minneapolis to San Diego and was given a room at University Hospital just a few floors above me. Dad, whose office was in the basement at that hospital, was relieved because it made it easier for him to check on each of us and keep an eye on our conditions.

Though he tried not to show it, he was increasingly worried, especially about me. "Dr. B was not an outwardly emotional person. He was very matter of fact about things," says longtime colleague Barbara Durrant. "But you could tell that all of his attention, all of his thinking, was focused on saving his son and caring for his daughter."

Dad went to Barbara and enlisted her in the cause, saying, "Rolf has to have surgery. He will likely need blood. Please see if you can get as many donors as possible."

Barbara did, donating blood herself and taking the request to colleagues and staff throughout the Zoo. "I was thrilled to be asked," Barbara says, "and happy that so many people agreed to give blood as well. We were, of course, all behind Dr. B. and Rolf and wanting to help however we could."

My surgery was scheduled for Saturday, October 13, but my body was not cooperating with that plan. When my anesthesiologist came to check on me on Friday night, my hands were trembling and sweat was beading on my forehead and running in rivulets down the sides of my face. My temperature and heart rate were way up, and my blood pressure was way down. The anesthesiologist recognized that I was experiencing septic shock. The planned surgery couldn't wait—I needed immediate help or I wouldn't make it to the morning.

The staff notified my surgeon, Dr. Gerald Peskin, who rushed to the hospital while I was being prepped. Once I was properly sedated, Dr. Peskin began the operation, removing 10 inches from my large intestine as well as a few inches from my small intestine. My parents were there at midnight when I was rolled out of surgery into the recovery room and then into the intensive care unit. They were grateful to hear that the operation had gone as well as it could have, given the circumstances.

The next morning, after checking on me, Dad went to his lab, where he knew the tissue removed from my body was waiting for his inspection. He gently pulled the tissue apart and was horrified by the extent of the lesions on the inside lining of the intestinal wall. "No wonder Rolf was in such pain," he thought. This was as bad as he'd ever seen.

Next, he placed slides of my colon under a microscope and peered through the lens. After a minute of close examination, he groaned.

"Something unusual, Kurt?" asked one of the technicians in the lab.

"Yes," Dad said. "I don't believe Rolf has Crohn's disease. These tissue samples are consistent with ulcerative colitis. I believe he may have been misdiagnosed." Dad knew that ulcerative colitis was a closely related inflammatory bowel disease (IBD), but one that affected the large intestine only. Though many of the treatments for ulcerative colitis were the same as those for Crohn's disease, some weren't, and Dad was concerned that my doctors had been addressing the wrong problem. It was another concern for our family in what seemed to be a never-ending ordeal.

A couple of days later, I heard the good news that Ingrid's kidney stone surgery had been successful and that she would be discharged from the hospital soon. But there was bad news as well. We learned that my mom's father—we called him "Opa"—was gravely ill in a hospital in Germany and was not expected to live long. Mom would need to fly out immediately to see him. Meanwhile, Dad was scheduled to leave in a few days to deliver an important keynote speech at a conference in Copenhagen, one that had been planned for over a year.

My parents wrestled with whether or not they should both leave us at such a critical time. I didn't make the decision any easier for them. I started having shakes, chills, and fever spikes every time the nurse had me try to get up for a short walk down the hall. Something was still wrong, but my doctors couldn't figure it out. Fortunately, my brother, Steve, was able to arrange to take time off from his medical school studies in Cleveland to fly out, support the family, and watch over Ingrid and me.

My fever started to subside a bit, so I urged my parents to take their trips.

The trips were important, and I was tired of being a burden. The next day, Mom and Dad both reluctantly headed to the airport and left on their flights, feeling at least encouraged that things were beginning to turn around for me.

Unfortunately, my recovery did not last. As my fourth week at University Hospital began, both my body and my spirit went downhill. Steve shared the news in a long-distance phone call five or six days later with Dad. "I'm afraid Rolf has taken a turn for the worse," Steve said. "There is concern that his bowel may be leaking somewhere into his abdomen, perhaps at the suture line where they reconnected the two ends of his intestines. The doctors think he may be turning septic, and something will have to be done . . . soon."

"Are they going to have to operate again?" Dad asked, concerned.

"Yes, and it may happen as soon as tomorrow. His fever's been going up and down like a yo-yo, especially after he gets out of bed and tries to take a walk of any kind. Right now, it's back up to 102 degrees, and he has those awful shaking chills again. The doctors are concerned he might have an abscess or a leak."

"My God, Steve!" Dad said. "Now I wish we hadn't gone! Mom will be very upset when she hears this." I can only imagine how helpless he must have felt at that moment, knowing he was over 5,000 miles away in Europe.

On October 26, eight days after my first operation, my doctors determined that I needed to go back into surgery. When they opened me up, their fears were confirmed. They found a small leak at the suture line right where the ileum (the final section of the small intestine) and the colon had been reconnected. The leak had enlarged into a bigger hole. The bacteria that normally lived inside my gut were now spilling into my abdomen and getting into my bloodstream. I was septic. The doctors knew they needed to act quickly, and creating an ileostomy was the only way to keep me alive. In an ileostomy, the surgeon takes the end of the small intestine and pulls it through a small incision made on a person's abdomen and fashions a stoma where an external pouch is attached to collect waste. In my case, the doctors also needed to create what's called a mucous fistula colostomy to anchor the colon that was left. There was no chance to explain this to me or anybody else. To give me the best chance of surviving, the doctors needed to finish this complex procedure as quickly as possible and get me on high doses of antibiotics.

Four hours after the operation started, the doctors sewed up my 10-inch abdominal incision with 13 heavy-gauge wire sutures that looked as barbaric as they felt. Somehow, I made it through the night, but when the anesthesia and pain medication began to wear off the next day, I was more shocked than grateful. Discovering that I'd ended up with an ileostomy and would be dealing with two stomas for the rest of my life was a hard reality to accept. A hundred thoughts flashed through my mind. What about my career and the sports I loved to play? Could I have a normal life? How could I do the things I loved with two appliances attached to my body? Nothing would ever be the same again. I was devastated.

My spirits were lifted the following day, however, when I heard Dad's authoritative, high-energy voice outside my room. He'd cut his Copenhagen trip short and flown home immediately after making his speech. "How's my son?" I heard him asking the nurses. A few moments later, he pulled back the curtain partition of my room in the ICU and walked over to my bed.

"Hi, Dad," I whispered through the discomfort of a tube stuck in my nose and down my throat. "It's great to see you."

"The feeling is mutual, Rolf," he said. He gently squeezed my hand. I later learned that over the previous few weeks at work, Dad had kept his emotions in check, admitting to his colleagues in a stoic tone, "We don't know if Rolf is going to make it." That didn't surprise me, as I could count on one hand the number of times that I'd seen him cry. Now, however, finding his son so weak and helpless, tears welled up in his eyes. As if a bit ashamed of this emotional display, my father turned away.

"It's okay, Dad," I said. Just knowing that he was back, that he cared so much, and that he was ready to take charge of the situation felt like the best news I'd had in a long, long time.

Later that day, he surprised me. Dad was in the room when Dr. Peskin, no doubt trying to raise my spirits, commented that he thought the Chargers were struggling without me. Dad spoke up: "The Chargers have won two games and lost one without Rolf. When he was with them in September, they were three and one. But they have missed him as a kicker. They're giving a new guy a try today. I can't think of his name."

"Mike Wood," I said, almost smiling. "Dad, I didn't know you followed the Chargers that closely."

"I read the sports page this morning," he said somewhat sheepishly. My father *never* read the sports section. It was the first time I'd seen him pay much attention to my football career, and it was uplifting.

Unfortunately, the next morning, October 29, my temperature spiked to 104 degrees again. I began to have hallucinations and nightmares, no doubt caused by the morphine I was given for the pain. My body was so weak by now that I felt I'd reached the end of my rope. I was sure I was dying.

Dad rushed back to the hospital as soon as he heard how badly I was doing. "Dad?" I asked.

"Yes, son?"

"I'm really scared." I squeezed my eyes shut for a moment. "Will you promise me one thing?"

"Yes. Whatever you want."

"Promise me that you won't let them keep me alive if there is no hope."

A long, agonizing silence settled between us. Finally, he spoke. "I promise. . . . I won't let them keep you alive that way."

Ingrid arrived at noon to visit, and Dad left my bedside for the first time in six hours. In the hallway outside the trauma unit, he ran into Bob Ortman, a longtime San Diego sportswriter who had quietly been stopping by the hospital almost every other day to get updates on my condition and pass me encouraging notes. He was of my dad's generation, another stoic who nevertheless felt things deeply, and someone I respected. For him to stop by as often as he did really touched me, especially since most of the time he wasn't even allowed to see me in the ICU.

"I hear he's in rough shape," Mr. Ortman said gently, seeing the pain in Dad's eyes.

Dad couldn't answer. All the pressure of the last two weeks had finally gotten the best of him. He began to sob big, heaving, body-shaking sobs. Mr. Ortman didn't hesitate—he wrapped his arms around Dad and let him cry.

That afternoon, my fever broke at last, and my body relaxed for the first time in 24 hours. Though I was weak, still in pain, and utterly exhausted, I was out of immediate danger. My body was finally ready to begin the process of healing.

I had a lot to learn about living with two small appliances—ostomy bags attached to my body—as well as more than a few doubts about whether I would ever feel "normal" again. But gradually, my health, attitude, and understanding of how to care for my appliances improved. As I slowly gained weight, I was allowed to return to the Chargers facility, where I was put in the capable hands of Phil Tyne, the team's strength coach, who helped nurse me back to health. Though I was pretty sure my NFL career was over, by June 1980 I was feeling like my old self. I had regained all of my weight and strength, and, except for the two appliances hanging on my sides, I felt pretty normal. When I asked Phil if he thought I'd ever be able to kick a football again, he looked at me as if I had two heads.

"What do you think we've been training so hard for?" Phil asked, almost indignantly. "Of course you can kick again! Let's go get some balls right now and kick a few so you can prove it to yourself."

A few minutes later, I found out that Phil was right. I *could* kick again. In fact, the ball was exploding off my foot. Even more importantly, the bags stayed secure and didn't get in the way. What had seemed like an impossible dream six months before was now actually a possibility. When training camp came around, I was given the green light by management to try out. Remarkably, I was able to earn my job back with the Chargers, becoming the first player in NFL history to play with an ostomy. How lucky was I?

I played for the Chargers for the next seven years and even made the Pro Bowl in 1982. Our team qualified for the playoffs for three straight years and played for the conference championship in 1981. Even more rewarding for me, however, was the opportunity that the NFL spotlight gave me to interact with and encourage people who were dealing with inflammatory bowel disease or an ostomy. It became a lifelong mission. During my worst moments in the hospital, I had expected to die—almost wished I would die—but I had been given a second chance to live and a second chance to play. It was a true blessing, and I wanted to make the most of it.

I experienced another unexpected blessing after my return to the NFL: Dad became an avid football fan. For the first time, he got into what I was doing and began attending my games. (Efficient as always, he was known to read a science journal between plays and during time-outs.) He even watched our games on TV when the Chargers were on the road and surprised me with his knowledge of what was going on in the league. Almost losing me and then seeing how hard I had to work to regain my job inspired most of that change, I'm sure. He realized how important playing football was to me. But he was also amazed by the response of the Chargers fan base. I had received sacks of mail from thousands of well-wishers while I was in the hospital. Many had told touching stories of their own struggles with IBD or other health issues. Nearly all of them had offered encouragement in some form, which meant more to me than I could ever express. Now that I had returned to the Chargers, people were contacting me to say how much I had encouraged and inspired them. My illness and recovery were resonating with many people.

One day Dad came to me and said in his usual straightforward tone, "Rolf, I don't really understand what you do, but you're clearly making a difference and I'm proud of you." By this point, I was feeling more comfortable in my own skin and less dependent on his approval. Even so, his words touched me deeply and were wonderful to hear.

Dad and I had much in common, but we were also different in many ways. Years later, I sent a letter to him using a car metaphor to explain how much I appreciated him, but how we had developed different approaches to life. The letter read, in part:

> Dad, when I was a kid growing up and you used to drive me and my buddies to hockey games or ski races, you used to drive really fast . . . in fact, so fast that my buddies were sometimes scared to get in the car with you. I was never scared, though, because I had great confidence in you. I knew you were a really good driver. You also always seemed to know where you were going, and that was always really comforting to me and to our whole family. But as I've grown up and learned to drive myself, I discovered that I drive differently than you. I don't drive as fast, and I don't always know where I'm going. It turns out that I like to explore the little "side streets" that life presents to us. I want you to know that you taught me how to drive, and I appreciate that, but I hope you'll also appreciate that I just drive a little differently.

Dad never acknowledged that letter. It may have stirred up too much emotion for him to bring it up with me directly. But Mom pulled me aside a few days later and said, "Dad got your letter, and it meant a lot to him. He *is* really proud of you."

Our relationship had changed over those difficult few years. I found myself not needing to prove anything to Dad anymore. I had become comfortable with who I was, and he had accepted me for me.

CHAPTER 19

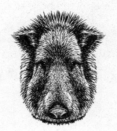

Proyecto Taguá

One of Dad's greatest passions and perhaps one of his proudest achievements began with, of all things, a bet. In the 1970s, on a trip to Paraguay, a University of Connecticut zoologist named Ralph Wetzel discovered a large peccary that had never been described in scientific literature. The peccary, a thin, piglike hoofed mammal with bristly, brown-gray fur, is native to Central and South America and the southwestern region of North America. But the animal that Wetzel came across was something new—much bigger and heavier, and, he later discovered, native only to Paraguay, Bolivia, and Argentina. Wetzel believed that this new species, now known as the giant Chacoan peccary (and locally as the *taguá*), was an ancestor of the extinct *platygonus* species of peccary.

When Dad met Wetzel at a conference and heard about the discovery, he was skeptical about Wetzel's theory. Dad suggested that the peccary might instead be a species that derived from *platygonus*; he didn't believe it was an ancestor. The two men couldn't agree. My father—annoyed to have his theory questioned—challenged Wetzel to a bet: $2,000, payable to the winner when further proof of the peccary's origins could be produced. Wetzel agreed.

To prove his hypothesis, Dad enlisted the help of an old acquaintance, Dennis Meritt, the assistant director of the Lincoln Park Zoo in Chicago at the time. (Dad always called him Charlie, though Dennis never knew why.)

Dennis tells the story of getting a call from my dad one day in 1980. "Charlie," the voice on the phone said, "I need your help. We're going on an expedition to Paraguay and Uruguay."

"Why would we do that?" Dennis asked quizzically.

"Well, I've made arrangements with the dictator of Paraguay, Alfredo Stroessner, to get a skin sample from a Chacoan peccary he has in their zoo, the only one held in a zoo in the world. We need to get a chromosome count so we can see how it compares to other peccaries. I need you to come with me, because you're going to immobilize the peccary at the zoo. I'm not sure how you're going to do that, but I know you'll figure it out."

Dennis had been to Paraguay twice before and had sworn he would never return. He'd found it nearly impossible to do fieldwork in the country's interior, because the forest—a dense combination of trees, thorny shrubs, cacti, and other prickly protuberances—was what the locals called "a living green hell." Nevertheless, this was Kurt Benirschke asking, one of the most fascinating, energetic, and knowledgeable men Dennis had ever met. How could he say no?

Dennis found himself boarding a plane in Miami with my dad, headed to Asunción in Paraguay. A day or two later, they presented themselves at the Botanical Garden and Zoo of Asunción, made arrangements with the staff, and were led to the rare Chacoan peccary. Dennis and two wildlife care staff members entered the large space, which was made up of shrubbery and a lot of dirt and dust, and they embarked on a merry chase to catch the peccary. When the staff members finally got ahold of it, they held the squirming animal while Dennis inserted a needle and injected an immobilization drug that he hoped was the proper dose to do the trick.

Dad, standing safely on the other side of the fence, called out, "Remember, Charlie, don't kill the pig! It's the dictator's peccary!" Still breathing hard from the chase and covered in dirt and mud, Dennis retorted, "No comments from the peanut gallery," and continued working.

The drug did its job. As soon as the peccary was asleep, Dad said, "Okay, Charlie, good work. I'll take it from here." My father, not completely sure how much time he had before the anesthetic wore off, quickly shaved and disinfected a section of the peccary's foreleg, took a small skin sample, and dropped it into a tube with tissue culture fluid.

Dad and Dennis thanked the staff for their help. Then they headed to a newly constructed biosafety lab on the outskirts of Asunción. Dad had arranged with the Paraguayan equivalent of the US Department of Agriculture to store his samples there while he and Dennis spent time in the country's interior.

The next day, they embarked on a six-hour bus trip to Dad's beloved Filadelfia, the German-speaking Mennonite community in the Chaco that he'd first visited in 1965. Over the next few days, they toured sites like the local hospital and natural history museum, shared meals and drinks at their hotel with the editor of Asunción's largest newspaper and his wife, and asked the locals for any information they knew about the Chacoan peccary. Dad also gave a long interview on the Filadelfia radio station—in German, of course.

It was a productive visit, but when it was time to leave, they faced a problem. Heavy rains were forecast for the next several days. It was illegal to travel on the clay-and-dirt Trans-Chaco Highway when it rained, because the water turned the road into a muddy quagmire, making it almost impassable. Getting stranded in Filadelfia would jeopardize their plans to obtain chromosome samples from another almost extinct animal, the La Plata river dolphin in Uruguay. It might even mean missing their flight home.

But Dad, ever industrious, found a solution. A local pilot was willing, for a fee, to fly the pair from Filadelfia to Asunción in his single-engine plane. Early the next morning, the pilot picked my dad and Dennis up at the hotel and drove them to the "airfield," a strip of dirt just outside of town that was surrounded by dense thorn forest. It was hot and sunny as they walked up to the tiny, rickety-looking aircraft. But enormous black storm clouds could be seen building in the sky to the south—exactly the direction they needed to go.

The plane had a pair of cockpit seats and another small jump seat behind them, which was where the luggage and supplies were stowed. "Charlie, you sit up front," Dad offered. "I really don't want to see what we're going to be flying into."

The pilot, a gregarious fellow with red hair and an optimistic disposition, didn't seem too worried. Once everyone settled in, the pilot taxied the plane southward and took off. Dennis held his breath as the plane just cleared the forest canopy and winged toward the ominous, dark mass of clouds ahead. The tiny craft was quickly engulfed by what seemed like a seething black monster ready to devour anything that dared to enter. Sudden downdrafts and violent upper air currents tossed the plane up and down. The pilot muttered something under his breath—Dennis later said, "I took enough German in high school to know it wasn't good"—and turned eastward.

"We can't go that way," the pilot said, shaking his head. "I think we'll try this way."

The small plane was no match for the churning storm. The pilot again muttered in German and maneuvered a complete about-face, this time pointing the plane west. Dennis swallowed and held onto the seat as tightly as he could. The plane rattled and shook; it felt like the plane might fall to pieces at any moment.

Dad, who'd been uncharacteristically silent up to this point, leaned forward from his seat in the back and yelled to Dennis over the roar of the engine, "Charlie, are we going to make it?"

"I am starting to pray!" Dennis replied.

The pilot, eyes ahead, had a determined expression. "We're going to punch through this!" he shouted. "Hang on!"

The turbulence continued as the tiny plane fought its way through the massive storm. The tense flight seemed to last forever, but it was just an hour later when the Asunción airport came into view. The three men let out a collective cheer, and Dad and Dennis slapped the pilot on the back. They had made it, surely cheating death. Following the landing, they stood grinning on the runway, shaking their heads. They'd never felt so grateful to be on solid ground.

Once they were back in Asunción, it was time to retrieve the peccary tissue cultures and head to Uruguay. However, it was a Saturday, and Dad and Dennis discovered that nobody worked on Saturdays. When they reached the modern, two-story brick edifice that served as the lab, a uniformed guard with a revolver on his hip crossed his arms and stood in front of the building, telling the scientists, "*Cerrado* [closed]."

They did their best to explain the situation and to persuade the guard to let them into the building, but to no avail. After more pestering and pleading, the guard finally agreed to find a phone (this was long before cell phones) and try to call someone who might give permission to the two crazy scientists. As soon as he saw the guard leave, Dad didn't hesitate.

"Come on," he said to Dennis. "Let's check around back and see if there's a way in." Sure enough, at the back of the lab, a window on the second floor was ajar.

"We've got to break in," Dad said. Dennis, who at age 42 was 16 years younger than Dad, realized that "we" meant him. Against his better judgment, Dennis was soon standing on my dad's back, trying to keep his balance as he stretched for the second-floor window ledge. He was desperately hoping not to slip—or be arrested and spend the rest of his days in a South American jail.

Dennis managed to curl his fingers around the ledge and haul himself up through the window and into the upstairs lab. Dad hurried to the front to serve as lookout in case the guard returned. Inside the lab, Dennis ignored the numerous yellow and red biohazard signs, located the room where the tissue cultures were kept, found what he was looking for, and slipped the containers into his pocket. Then he snuck downstairs to the locked front door and let himself out. He found Dad waiting for him just outside.

A moment later, the guard returned. Dennis had made it with just seconds to spare. Dad calmly walked to the front door, pushed down on the handle, and feigned surprise when the door opened.

"Oh," he said to the guard, "you don't have to call anybody after all. The door's unlocked." The guard looked confused but fortunately asked no questions.

Just then, a vehicle pulled up to the front of the lab. The lab's director got out and apologized for the confusion. He led the two men into the building to the room where the tissue cultures were stored. Dad and Dennis had to pretend they were obtaining the cultures they had already taken, or they'd risk being caught. They did take advantage of the extra time to add fresh tissue fluid to the cultures for the long trip home. The director, apparently none the wiser and intent on making amends, produced a bottle of Scotch and served everyone fried chicken and drinks for lunch. The near disaster turned into a party—and another adventure story.

"Every time I think of that day, I think about all the things that could have gone wrong," Dennis recalls with a chuckle. "But to Kurt, it was what had to be done. [It was] logical as far as he was concerned—and those cultures were invaluable. Besides, I was convinced that if something bad had happened to us, Kurt would've just talked our way out of it, as I've seen him do countless other times."

At their hotel that evening, the hotel owner, a German national known as Herr Wagner, treated Dad and Dennis to an elegant dinner. Halfway through a bottle of wine, my father suddenly looked Dennis in the eye and said, "Charlie, we've got to do something here for the Chacoan peccary. This is important. I don't know exactly what we should do yet, but I think we can get the San Diego Zoo involved, and we'll figure it out." The Chacoan peccary was critically endangered. If someone didn't take action, the animal would soon be extinct. They made a pact that evening to create a Chacoan peccary rescue and conservation plan and present it to the San Diego Zoo.

After returning to the United States, Dad was eager to examine his new tissue samples. He discovered that the Chacoan peccary had only 20 chromosomes, far fewer than the 30 chromosomes of the collared peccary and the 26 of the white-lipped peccary. Dad was right: the Chacoan peccary had derived from the *platygonus,* rather than the other way around. He was excited to share the news with Ralph Wetzel and collect on his bet. But sadly, Ralph Wetzel passed away soon after the test results were known, before Dad could connect with him.

My father was now on a mission. With the endorsement and cooperation of the International Union for Conservation of Nature (IUCN), he and Dennis made good on their pact and created a Species Survival Plan for the Chacoan peccary. Dad enlisted support for the plan from San Diego Zoo officials. In November 1983, he returned to the Chaco and, with his own funds, bought a piece of property in the forest west of Filadelfia that included a former Mennonite schoolhouse. His vision was to turn it into a peccary breeding center.

In 1985, he returned again, this time with his assistant Mary (Byrd) Cole, who spoke Spanish, and researcher Arlene Kumamoto in tow. On these trips and via long-distance coordinating, they refurbished the one-story schoolhouse, purchased peccaries from locals who kept them as pets or for food, and employed a series of helpers. The first was a volunteer from the Peace Corps who caught Dad's excitement and served as the local liaison. The new "ranch" was rustic, featuring an open kitchen and a fenced backyard made up of dense brush and feeding stations for the peccaries. But it was a start. They established a breeding colony of animals and, starting in 1985, Dennis Meritt made nearly annual trips back to the Chaco to manage the conservation program.

Sometime after their 1985 trip, Dad approached Mary back at the Zoo. "You know," he said with a twinkle in his eye, "someone needs to go back to Paraguay and find out more about these peccaries."

Mary, sitting at her desk, just laughed. "Yeah, where are you going to find someone to do that?"

When my dad grinned, Mary realized she'd been had. "I think," he said, "that would be a great thing for *you* to do." An adventurer at heart and someone who loved a challenge, Mary agreed.

In April 1986, she found herself traveling solo back to Paraguay, excited but a bit apprehensive about this new adventure. She spent much of the next two years in the Chaco coordinating the peccary conservation program, known locally as *Proyecto Taguá*.

It was not always a comfortable existence. "I was surprised I stayed alive down there," Mary says today with a wry smile. "The first thing I did was tell the local people that I was there to work with animals and that I had nothing to do with the CIA. If the drug smugglers thought you were CIA, they'd kill you. If you were on one of their cocaine roads and in the way, you were gone. I never went anywhere without a rifle." Another concern was the possibility of encountering one of the many venomous snakes in the forest. On one of their outings, Dad asked Mary, "How come when we're here, you always walk in front of me?"

"Because the first person on the trail wakes the snakes up," she explained with a chuckle, "but they don't bite until the second person comes along."

Despite the risks, the program flourished. By the end of 1986, the population had grown to nearly 70 animals, necessitating that some be released back into their native habitat.

In November of that year, Dad returned to check in on Mary and the peccary program. While they were there, they received a surprise invitation to a formal Thanksgiving dinner at the American embassy in Buenos Aires. It turned out that the ambassador had family in San Diego and had learned about what the Zoo was doing with the peccaries; he wanted to thank Dad. My father hadn't packed any dress clothes, so he showed up at the formal event in a casual, untucked guayabera shirt, his customary high-water slacks, and Rockport tennis shoes. Everyone else was decked out in their finest dinner attire. But Dad wasn't the least bothered and thoroughly enjoyed the evening.

Some things could unsettle him, however. One involved his first night in the Chaco on that 1986 visit. When Dad arrived, Mary gave up her usual bedroom in the refurbished schoolhouse to sleep in another room with Gina, the Peace Corps volunteer. Dad was exhausted from his travels and ready for some rest. In the bedroom, he got undressed, arranged the curtains around the bed that screened out bugs, and crawled in. What he didn't know was that one of the first peccaries that Mary and Gina had brought in from their native habitat, a young female they'd named Melinda, had bonded with Mary. During the day, Melinda followed Mary wherever she went in the house. In the evening, she followed Mary into the bedroom and squealed until Mary picked her up and put her at the foot of the bed where she would sleep—that is, until Melinda grew big enough to jump into the bed by herself.

Mary and Gina were just settling down to sleep when they heard a sudden series of exclamations, thrashing, and stomps from the other bedroom. A moment later, Dad burst into their room, wild-eyed and disheveled, wearing only his shorts.

"There's something in my bed!" he shrieked.

When she was finally able to stop laughing, Mary explained her "sleeping arrangement" with the young peccary. "You're just going to have to sleep with her like that," she said with a smile, "because that animal knows that's where she sleeps." To Dad's credit, he did adjust to sharing a bed with his unexpected nighttime partner.

On the same trip, Dad, Mary, and Gina were walking in the forest after a hard rain when Dad felt something wriggling inside one of his boots. He hurriedly sat down on a rock, yanked off the boot, and started cussing. "Leeches!" he shrieked. "Help me get 'em off! Help me get 'em off! I can feel them munching on me!" Mary and Gina couldn't help laughing at their usually stoic leader's discomposure.

Despite these occasional misadventures, my dad absolutely loved Paraguay and the Chaco. The German-speaking Mennonites and their familiar and tasty meals were a heartwarming reminder of his youth. The wildness of the region also appealed to him. In the evenings, he often sat on the screened front porch of the schoolhouse, smoking a pipe and simply taking in the sounds of the Chaco. Once in a while, after a day of working with peccaries and making new friends among the Paraguayans, he would set up a hammock on the porch and sleep there for the night.

Dad even talked about retiring in the Chaco, but Mom had no interest in that. He did persuade her to make one trip to Paraguay. Although she was a good sport about it, one trip was enough for her.

During one off-season in the 1980s when I was still playing for the Chargers, I made my own trip to Paraguay with Dad and with Mary's son, Chris, who was about my age. I was especially impressed by the industriousness of the Filadelfians, who had literally carved a self-sustaining existence out of a place that most people would consider uninhabitable. I got to work with the peccaries, did a lot of bird-watching, rode horses with Chris, and watched him put his artistic talents to work when he painted a sign for the entrance to the ranch that read, "*Proyecto Taguá*." Like Mom, I didn't see Paraguay as a place I'd want to live on a permanent basis. But I understood Dad's passion for the country and its inhabitants, both human and nonhuman, and the rugged beauty of the Chaco.

∞

In 1995, Dad made a phone call to Dennis Meritt, who was still working for the Lincoln Park Zoo at the time. In a distressed voice, he explained that the leadership at the San Diego Zoo decided it could no longer support expenses for peccary conservation because the funds were needed for other projects. He couldn't afford to take on those expenses himself. Now, the future of the project and the Chacoan peccary was on the line. Would Dennis be willing to take over as project leader and fundraiser?

Dennis agreed. He recruited people to work on-site in the Chaco and solicited funds from representatives who had added or hoped to add Chacoan peccaries to their zoos. Dad decided to donate the Chaco property he had purchased to the on-site project managers. The property was sold, and the conservation team purchased land and a house adjacent to the original ranch house. With my father's consistent encouragement and support, Dennis kept the conservation program going, and they both continued to visit Paraguay and the Chaco.

Today, the conservation program in the Chaco includes two ranch houses, one for the daily staff and one for visiting scientists. More than 100 Chacoan peccaries continue to live on-site, and another estimated 75 peccaries have been exported and now reside in zoos in North America and Europe. Interestingly, it was Melinda, Mary's faithful peccary companion and Dad's bedmate for a few nights, who became the matriarch of this line of peccaries.

Although Chacoan peccaries are still listed as endangered, several hundred have been released into their native habitat, enough to create a self-sustaining population. In addition, the government of Paraguay has set aside roughly 400 acres as a wildlife preserve for a host of animals, including the peccary. The ranch houses, Chacoan peccary colony, and wildlife preserve are now maintained by a nongovernmental organization, the Chaco Center for Conservation and Research. Dennis remains highly involved and returns to Paraguay at least once a year to check in with the full-time veterinarian in Paraguay who serves as the program's executive director. *Proyecto Taguá* is still the world's only conservation management program for the Chacoan peccary. The program saved this unique animal and continues to act as the primary hedge against the species' extinction.

On one trip to the Chaco, Dennis got to spend time with a trio of Paraguayan veterinary students who were working at the ranch to fulfill a fieldwork requirement for their schooling. On their first day, the students learned how to immobilize the peccaries and then do a complete physical on the animals. Up to that point in their training, they had spent very little time treating wildlife and were understandably tentative. By the third day, however, they were confidently moving about the yard and performing the procedures without assistance, thrilled by what they were learning.

"As I watched these students," Dennis recalls, "I thought about how good Kurt would have felt if he'd been there and seen them. The program that he envisioned, and we committed to build together, is continuing to do what we intended. Not only is it saving the Chacoan peccary, but it has also become an asset to the country and its people."

None of this would have been possible without Dad's vision and passion for an animal on the verge of extinction.

"What Kurt did in the Chaco for peccaries," Dennis says, "is the perfect example of the saying, 'Anything is possible when you put your mind to it.' Kurt demonstrated that countless times, to me and to everyone who knew him."

CHAPTER 20

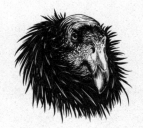

SAVING WILDLIFE

Directly and indirectly, Dad influenced numerous efforts to protect and revitalize endangered wildlife all over the planet. One of the most significant was the drive to save the California condor.

This majestic bird, with a wingspan of nearly 10 feet and capable of soaring as fast as 55 miles per hour, is the largest bird in North America. Thousands of years ago, the condor could be found in ranges across the continent. Human population growth, however, reduced the condor's habitat and food sources. The condor population was also nearly wiped out by ingesting carrion that contained lead bullets and consuming poisons meant to control other animal populations. By 1980, the California condor was on the brink of extinction. Only 22 birds remained in the world, their habitat limited to mountainous regions of Southern California east of Santa Barbara.

At the San Diego Zoo, a team of board members and committee members consisting of my dad, executive staff and managers, and wildlife care specialists met with government, education, and zoological agencies. After a lot of discussion, they formed a plan. They agreed that the only chance the birds had was if all the remaining California condors were captured and brought into zoos for safety. The plan was controversial, but ultimately, two facilities, the San Diego Wild Animal Park and the Los Angeles Zoo, were selected to house the birds.

The next challenge was determining how to catch the birds, which nested in remote mountains that were difficult to reach. The condor team decided to try to lure them to the ground by setting bait near known nesting sites. The team then dug holes in the ground big enough for a person to sit in, covered the hole with leaf-filled tree limbs, and laid a goat carcass on top. A lucky Zoo intern was then given the job of crawling into the hole, hiding, and waiting . . . often for hours. When a soaring condor eventually spied the dead goat and settled on it to feed, the intern had to reach up through the tree limbs, grab the condor by the legs, and hold on long enough for the other team members—who were hiding in nearby bushes—to throw nets over the huge bird and subdue it. (I have great admiration for the dedication of those interns. Waiting in a dark hole for who knows how long in the California heat, enduring flies and the smell of the dead goat, and braving the talons of an unhappy condor was not a job many people wanted!)

Half the condors were sent to the Wild Animal Park's new "Condorminium" and half were sent to the Los Angeles Zoo, with males and females at each facility. Most condors choose long-term mates, so the team knew it was extremely important to select the right partner for maximum breeding potential. In the early days, the team took a blood sample of a newly arrived condor. The sample was then flown by helicopter to the Zoo's research lab where cytogenetics specialist Arlene Kumamoto completed chromosome tests to determine the condor's sex. According to federal regulations, a condor could be kept in temporary quarters for only 48 hours before it had to be assigned to its permanent home or released. Arlene figured out how to speed up the testing process to accommodate the rules.

Once the gender was known, the condor was paired with another condor either at the Los Angeles Zoo or at the Wild Animal Park.

The effort to place California condors under human care began in 1982, but it wasn't until 1987 that the last wild condor was brought in. No one knew if the well-intended breeding program would succeed, especially since condors usually lay only one egg a year. But once the program's first condor chick hatched in 1988, the birds began producing offspring steadily.

The team figured out how to increase the number of chicks hatched each year by using a method called double-clutching. A condor pair's first egg was hatched in an incubator and hand-reared using a condor puppet so the chick wouldn't imprint on its human caregivers. Then the condors produced a second egg and raised that chick themselves, thus doubling the number of chicks a pair could produce each season. The goal was to reintroduce adult condors into their native habitat. In 1992, this work paid off when the team released the first two zoo-bred condors. This milestone day demonstrated what could be accomplished when different agencies, authorities, scientists, and zoos worked together on a common mission.

Today, although the California condor is still listed as critically endangered and its future is far from secure, it is clearly making a comeback, thanks to the breeding program. Nearly 20 chicks hatch each year at what has now expanded to four breeding centers, including the original site at the former Wild Animal Park (now the San Diego Zoo Safari Park). Birds have also been released in Central California, Southern California, Arizona, and Baja California, Mexico. As of 2022, the number of condors has grown from what was once a world population of just 22 birds to more than 500, with just under 340 soaring in the wild. The California condor program is now a model for other conservation efforts.

Another high-profile conservation program that involved my dad and the conservation research team at the San Diego Zoo was the international effort to save the giant panda. Native to China, the popular black-and-white bears live a mostly isolated existence, feasting on bamboo in damp, misty forests. Between 1974 and 1985, however, logging and other human encroachment eliminated half of the available panda habitats, and the situation became dire. The giant panda's numbers in the wild dropped to less than 1,000, and it was listed as endangered.

In 1989, the Chinese Ministry of Forestry and the World Wildlife Fund formulated a management plan for the giant panda and its habitat. Despite this effort, no one knew if pandas could be saved from extinction. Little research had been done on their behavior in the wild, and pandas were not reproducing well in zoos. In the 1990s, the Chinese government reached out to officials at the San Diego Zoo to see if they would be willing to help. A partnership quickly developed between the Zoo and its Chinese colleagues to create a breeding strategy. It was a natural alliance, in part because two giant pandas had been loaned to the Zoo in 1987 and a good relationship had already begun to form.

Doug Myers, then executive director of the Zoological Society of San Diego (now San Diego Zoo Wildlife Alliance), and Don Lindburg, the wildlife behaviorist my father hired in 1979 to join the conservation research department, were part of the team that completed a complex, unprecedented, multiyear negotiation with the China Wildlife Conservation Association to bring two giant pandas to the San Diego Zoo in 1996.

The hope was that the two pandas, Bai Yun and Shi Shi, would produce offspring. Unfortunately, that didn't happen. The male, Shi Shi, showed no interest in mating with Bai Yun, much to the disappointment of everyone at the Zoo. Officials later discovered that Shi Shi was much older than originally believed. More importantly, they learned that Shi Shi's pheromone receptor, which males depend upon to pick up the scent of an ovulating female, might have been damaged in a fight with another male in the wild. Although Bai Yun showed all the signs that she was ready to mate, Shi Shi didn't seem to notice. To make matters even more challenging, research showed that giant panda females were receptive to breeding only two or three days per year. If this very narrow window was missed, everyone would have to wait another year!

Upon learning all of this, the Zoo's team members took matters into their own hands, deciding to try artificial insemination techniques they had been developing. This was a big decision—artificial insemination had never been tried with giant pandas before, and the process required all the cumulative knowledge the team had been gathering to that point about the hormones, cycles, and reproductive behavior of pandas. Once the protocols were determined, Barbara Durrant, head of reproductive sciences, impregnated Bai Yun with sperm collected from Shi Shi and the team waited. To everyone's excitement and relief, it worked! The Zoo's first cub, Hua Mei, entered the world in 1999. She was also the first panda born in the United States that survived and grew into adulthood.

This huge accomplishment led to the construction of the Giant Panda Research Station and the giant panda habitat at the Zoo, under Don Lindburg's leadership. Don and the team also began working with their Chinese colleagues to find a younger male panda that was capable of natural breeding.

Unfortunately, the Zoo's contract with China stipulated that a replacement could be offered only if one of the original pandas died. In a meeting with officials in Beijing, Don approached the issue with a creative and daring strategy. As they discussed the contract, Don said, "Well—why don't we declare Shi Shi dead?"

This was unexpected. Don recalls that the Chinese scientists "were scratching their heads, laughing a little bit, and looking at each other. Finally, they said, 'Okay.' That was a big moment for us—it showed that both sides were all in to get something done."

Still very much alive, Shi Shi was successfully shipped back to China to live out his elder years. His replacement in January 2003 was Gao Gao, a healthy, inquisitive young male that did, indeed, breed with Bai Yun. Mei Sheng, a male cub, was born later that year, the second of six cubs that Bai Yun gave birth to in San Diego. With each new birth, scientists gained more knowledge, furthering the reproductive and behavioral science and providing hope for panda conservation.

The Zoo did much more than produce offspring to increase the population of giant pandas during this partnership with China. The Zoo staff also developed early-detection pregnancy tests, ultrasound procedures, and a milk formula for panda cubs that dramatically increased survival rates. Staff members learned how important it was to allow a new mother and her cub to be alone and bond for the first several months after birth. In addition, researchers began using GPS technology to track pandas in the wild so they could learn how far the wildlife ranged. In 2010, the giant panda reached a major milestone, with 300 pandas in zoos and breeding centers. Researchers believed there was enough genetic diversity to ensure a healthy, self-sustaining population. For my father and fans of the giant panda, it was a tremendous success story.

As I witnessed the exciting developments and successes taking place in conservation, I wanted to come up with my own way to help save endangered wildlife and support Dad's continuing research for the Zoo. As an NFL player, I had a platform and the opportunity to direct attention to something that could make a difference. The agent who negotiated my football contracts, Leigh Steinberg, was young and idealistic and would become one of the best and most creative agents in the business. In 1980, we came up with a campaign we called Kicks for Critters. I pledged to contribute money for every field goal I kicked in a game to support the conservation efforts at the Zoo. At the same time, I encouraged the people of San Diego to join me and donate whatever dollar amount they could with every successful kick I made. The idea caught on, and thousands of people pledged their support.

It was satisfying to put my football career to work for something that meant a lot to me personally. It was also fun to give Dad another reason to keep up on my games—I knew he was now rooting for me in more ways than one!

While the program we started has morphed, it is still going strong. Today it is an annual fundraising event held at the Zoo every fall. Now known as the San Diego Zoo Food, Wine & Brew Celebration, it is typically attended by about 3,000 people.

In addition to Kicks for Critters, I started the Cans for Critters program in grade schools around San Diego with help from the fundraising team and a blessing from the Zoo's director at the time, Chuck Bieler. Kids learned about endangered wildlife while collecting and recycling aluminum cans and then donating the proceeds to the Zoo. More than 100 schools were involved, and kids all over the city learned about the importance of recycling and the challenges facing wildlife. By 1987, we had raised more than $1.5 million for the Center for Reproduction of Endangered Species (CRES) and helped draw even more attention to the plight of endangered wildlife.

Perhaps Dad's most unusual conservation project began in a New York bar. His book about the placenta had made him the first US author for Springer-Verlag's New York book publishing division. In 1984, he was invited to give the after-dinner speech at the 20th anniversary celebration of the company. His talk was, naturally, about endangered wildlife. Publisher Heinz Götze, who had become a personal friend of Dad's, also invited the famous and eccentric artist Andy Warhol.

After the talk, Dad, Götze, and Warhol retired to the bar together for a celebratory drink. They were a surprising trio—a publisher, a world-renowned pathologist, and a leading figure in the American pop art movement. As they talked, Götze proposed an idea that he clearly had been thinking about for a while: would Warhol create art for a book written by my father about endangered wildlife? It was, Dad later wrote, "easier to persuade me to do this than it was to get Andy's consent." But by the end of the evening, all were in agreement.

At Dad's suggestion, the trio planned to feature 15 endangered animals that weren't in the public eye at the time but were important to him, including the Sumatran rhinoceros, whooping crane, douc langur, okapi, California condor, and of course the giant Chacoan peccary. The plan was for my dad to write the text and Warhol to provide the art. Dad sent Warhol photographs of the animals in different positions—twice, just to make sure he received them. Dad and Heinz Götze also made more than one visit to the Factory, Warhol's New York studio, to work on the book. The inspired book, *Vanishing Animals,* was released in 1986. It received critical praise and became a collector's item.

Some people, Mom included, were surprised to hear that Dad would collaborate with a controversial character like Andy Warhol. But to Dad, it was a great opportunity to reach an entirely different group of people and educate them about the plight of endangered wildlife. The book raised awareness of relatively unknown wildlife in danger of extinction and helped him raise money for the conservation research at the Zoo. It also validated Heinz Götze's vision of what this unusual pair could do together. I proudly display the book on my coffee table to this day.

CHAPTER 21

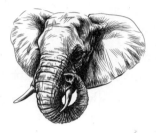

PRESIDENT BENIRSCHKE

By 1985, Dad had presided over the Zoo's conservation research effort for a decade. He watched it grow from an uncertain, fledgling enterprise into a scientific force with a growing international reputation. As he wrote in the 1984 *CRES Annual Report*, "When the board accepted the white papers of the research council which created a division of research, it probably had no inkling what a thorny plant it was to chew on. Research in zoos was antithetical, and it has been a long effort to convince all parties of the necessity to have research." Yet in 10 years, the case had been made. Dad had spoken at conferences around the world, repeatedly extolling the need for zoo conservation research and relating the positive difference it was making. The San Diego Zoo staff had published 246 scientific papers, 47 abstracts, 50 book chapters, 7 books, and 46 popular articles—an astounding amount of research. The conservation research department had become a legitimate part of the Zoo. Other zoos around the globe were also, formally or informally, initiating and expanding their own research efforts. Zoo-based wildlife conservation research was here to stay.

Dad was now ready for a change in responsibilities. He'd been invited to join the Zoo's board of trustees, a prestigious position that would in some ways give him even greater influence over the Zoo's research and conservation efforts. At age 61, he wasn't even close to being ready to slow down. "Slow" wasn't in my father's DNA. His duties at the university were also expanding. He was now UCSD's director of autopsy services, and he continued to juggle his medical school teaching responsibilities and his role in the pathology department. He was also eager to write what he felt was a long-overdue second edition of his textbook *Pathology of the Human Placenta*.

In 1986, Dad joined the Zoo's board of trustees and stepped down as director of research. Werner Heuschele, who'd earned his doctorate in medical microbiology and had come to the Zoo in 1981, was named to succeed Dad. Of course, my father continued to make multiple visits every week to the Scripps building to check on projects, work with staff, and encourage their progress. Everyone knew when he was on site—the familiar aroma of his special blend of pipe tobacco always wafted throughout the building.

Marlys Houck, a cytogenetics specialist who initially came to the Zoo in 1987 on a one-year grant to develop cell lines of the critically endangered northern white rhino, remembers one of her first meetings with my dad. Late one evening, she and Arlene Kumamoto were walking downstairs to leave for the day. Dad had just arrived—you never knew when he might pop in—and he was bounding up the stairs, pipe clenched in his teeth. They met on the landing between floors, where he asked about another project Marlys was working on.

"Have you done the chromosomes for the Sumatran rhino yet?" Dad asked.

"No," Marlys said, shaking her head. "I'm having trouble getting the chromosomes to spread."

Dad asked a few more questions and made several helpful suggestions. As they talked, both of them began to see new possibilities.

"It had been a long day," Marlys recalls, "and I had really been looking forward to going home. But Dr. B was so enthusiastic, and the more we talked, the more we both got excited. By the end of our conversation, I wanted to run back upstairs and go back to work. He was just so inspiring."

That same year, Dad took a six-month sabbatical from UCSD to work on the new edition of his pathology textbook. Up to this point, he had written all of his papers and manuscripts on a typewriter, using just two fingers in his "hunt and peck" style. For years, colleagues had urged him to use a computer to speed up the process, but he had never taken the time to learn how one worked. That finally changed when Dad walked into a store and purchased his first computer. From there, he never looked back.

He learned software programs and wrote, with coauthor Peter Kaufmann, a completely new placenta volume, nearly 900 pages long, on his new computer. Every few years after that, Dad upgraded his personal computer and laptop to a newer and faster machine, donating his old one to one of us kids. As was so often the case, he made himself an expert in this area too and introduced the latest technology to our family and his younger colleagues.

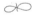

Dad's next few years included continuing progress in multiple areas of research and conservation, as well as considerable travel, especially trips to the Chaco in Paraguay to check on the peccaries. But even my indefatigable father could not keep going at that pace, as we all came to realize the night of January 7, 1993.

He was at an upscale San Diego restaurant, preparing to host a group of friends for dinner and conversation, when he suddenly felt pain in his chest and forearms and began to perspire. When the first guest arrived, he asked her to take over hosting the group and to call for an ambulance. At the hospital, tests confirmed his suspicions—he was having a heart attack. After a balloon angioplasty and nearly a week in the hospital, Dad recovered and was sent home with orders to reduce stress in his life—including to stay away from his offices and labs for the next two months. He responded to this directive in his typical fashion: "I'm crushed. But then, I could also have died, and this is better."

The heart attack, combined with changes at the university and a long list of projects he hadn't had time to get to, led Dad to an important decision—he would retire from the university the following summer, at 70 years old. His retirement party in 1994 was a festive affair attended by 200 well-wishers. A highlight was the announcement that the university would sponsor an annual Kurt Benirschke lecture featuring international experts on topics relevant to biology and reproduction, as well as a Kurt Benirschke fellowship in reproductive pathology. At the party, Steve, Ingrid, and I read aloud from a large collection of notes that friends and colleagues had written to Dad. He later wrote, "That brought forth wonderful responses and much nostalgia of the past. So many friends came from so many places. I was simply overwhelmed."

For Dad, of course, retirement hardly meant sitting at home and watching TV. As a professor emeritus, he still maintained an office at UCSD and went to his lab every day. He also continued to work with colleagues at the Zoo, staying as involved as ever—just not getting paid for it. In 1997, the board of trustees recognized his commitment by voting to make him president of the Zoological Society of San Diego (president of the board of trustees), effective January 1, 1998. It was a humbling responsibility. Dad was now charged with leading the board of trustees and setting the future course for both the Zoo and the Wild Animal Park. (His three-year term as president had an inauspicious start, however. On the last day of 1997, the admissions staff member at the entrance to the Wild Animal Park didn't believe he was the new president and initially refused to let him in!)

With the beginning of the New Year, there was a flurry of meetings and projects at the Zoo that left no doubt changes were afoot. New features at the Zoo that started during my father's presidency and were completed over the next several years included an upgrade and expansion of the gorilla habitat; the opening of Ituri Forest, a replica of an African rainforest featuring hippos, monkeys, okapis, otters, and forest buffalo; a renovation of Owens Aviary; and a new home for red river hogs. Improvements at the Wild Animal Park included the opening of Condor Ridge and the construction of a new bird breeding center. The Zoo and thousands of daily visitors celebrated the groundbreaking births of three Malayan tiger cubs, two Chacoan peccaries from mothers that had arrived from Paraguay, and one giant panda—Hua Mei—born via artificial insemination in 1999, an event heralded around the world.

One of Dad's greatest achievements during his tenure as president was persuading the board of trustees to join him on a trip to visit Europe's best zoos. In May 1999, he chaperoned a party of 18 board members and their spouses on a tour of 15 of the world's oldest and most famous zoos. They stopped in London, Paris, Zurich, and the German cities of Cologne, Leipzig, and Berlin, where they toured Zoo Berlin and Tierpark Berlin. According to Doug Myers, then executive director and CEO of San Diego Zoo Global, the 11-day trip was grueling: "We were on a plane, a train, a bus, in a zoo, and then back on a plane. But it was also an amazing and unforgettable experience."

All reports indicate the group had a great time. Even more important from my dad's perspective, however, was that he and the other board members had a chance to see firsthand what other zoos were doing well. The trip expanded the board members' understanding of what was possible in San Diego. They returned home with a host of new ideas to consider . . . feeling fully energized and a little worn out!

During Dad's presidency, he had to make a difficult decision about elephant breeding. The popularity of pachyderms made them a natural choice for zoos. The San Diego Zoo's first pair of elephants had arrived in 1923, but with the challenges of breeding elephants—females typically deliver an offspring once every four years—the first elephant birth for the organization wasn't until 1981 at the Wild Animal Park. Despite the difficulties, other zoos across the country had slowly become more successful with breeding elephants. By the 1990s, zoos had run out of space for more elephants and most decided to stop breeding them altogether. Then a study in 2000 showed that the population of elephants in North American zoos was dying out. Unless breeding resumed, fewer than 20 would remain in these zoos by 2050.

The decision of whether or not to emphasize breeding again was made more challenging by animal rights groups that argued against keeping elephants in zoos. In addition, elephants were considered to be among the most dangerous animals to manage, and they required a long-term commitment that some zoos couldn't make. As Dad said, "When you decide to breed elephants, you have to think 200 years into the future." After a lot of thought and discussion, he and the board ultimately chose to endorse a renewed elephant breeding program at the Wild Animal Park, believing it was the way zoos could help ensure the species' survival for the long term.

As president, Dad was also looking ahead when he proposed hosting an international conference to explore the benefits and options for conserving the genetic heritage of life on Earth and what role the Frozen Zoo might play. He used his connections and influence to assemble a stellar group of speakers and experts on reproduction that included Ian Wilmut, an English embryologist and pioneer in the cloning of animals; Francis Crick, a codiscoverer of DNA's double helix structure and Nobel Prize winner; and Sydney Brenner, a molecular biologist and Nobel Prize winner. Ollie Ryder organized the May 2000 conference, titled "Genetic Resources for the New Century." Though the conservation world was not yet ready to embrace all the ideas and options presented by the Frozen Zoo and similar efforts, the gathering did advance conservationists' thinking about what was possible.

Perhaps the most significant event during my father's presidency occurred in January 2000 when the Arnold and Mabel Beckman Foundation announced a $7.5 million grant to the Zoo to help build a conservation research center on the grounds of the Wild Animal Park. The state-of-the-art, 50,000-square-foot Arnold and Mabel Beckman Center for Conservation Research, completed in 2004, featured offices, a library, a conference room, and 20,000 square feet of laboratory space that would include the Frozen Zoo. Dad's vision for animal research had found a permanent and well-designed home in San Diego. The Beckman Center for Conservation Research remains the largest zoo-based, multidisciplinary conservation research and science facility in the world.

As the year 2000 came to an end, so did Dad's role as president of the board. He looked back with satisfaction at the board's many achievements from the previous three years, yet he also felt relieved about letting someone else carry the responsibility for a while. He was ready to devote more time to personal projects, including a comparative placentation website. That site grew to include more than 50 species, with each entry offering general zoological data, images, genetic analysis, and detailed information about the characteristics of each animal's placenta and reproductive process. It became one of the world's most important resources for comparative placentation of animals and is still available today (placentation.ucsd.edu).

At the start of 2001, at age 76, Dad was as curious and excited as ever about life and scientific discoveries that were still waiting to be made. One of the most promising arenas to explore was the field of genetics and how advances there might be applied to wildlife conservation.

CHAPTER 22

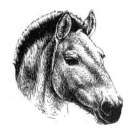

NEW HOPE

On a Monday morning, February 24, 1997, Ollie Ryder burst into my father's office in the research building at the Zoo. "Did you hear about Dolly the sheep?" he asked excitedly. "This isn't supposed to be possible. It can't be!"

Dad grinned, knowing exactly what Ollie was talking about. "Well," he said, "now we know that it *is* possible."

That weekend, news stations had reported that a few months earlier, a team of scientists in Scotland had created the world's first successfully cloned mammal from an adult cell. The scientists had taken the nucleus from an adult sheep cell, transferred it into an unfertilized egg, stimulated the hybrid cell with an electric shock, and then implanted it into a surrogate sheep mother. The birth of Dolly the sheep caused a sensation. It showed that an adult cell could be "rebooted"—meaning that DNA from an adult cell could be used to develop an entirely new organism, dispelling the decades-long assumption that adult mammals could not be cloned.

"There are so many possibilities of how we could apply this here at the Zoo," Dad said with enthusiasm. He was on his way out of the office to a meeting, so Ollie walked with him.

"No doubt. We really need to explore the animal conservation implications of this," Ollie said.

"Let's write a paper about it," Dad suggested.

"You bet," Ollie answered.

"Okay," Dad said, "I'll get it started." Within a week, they were ready to submit "The Potential Use of 'Cloning' in the Conservation Effort" to the science journal *Zoo Biology*. Their paper stated that "cloning cannot replace current practices of preservation of wild animals" but that "the potential rewards are considerable" and that cloning had "the potential of minimizing loss of genetic resources as well as rescuing already lost genetic material; these may be its greatest assets."

Despite the possibilities, cloning was controversial in many quarters. Some people feared the potential misuse of this new technology for both humans and animals. They may have had in mind the 1993 blockbuster movie *Jurassic Park*, which portrayed cloning experiments with dinosaurs that went awry. Interestingly, Dad's research team had its own connection to that movie. Before filming began, an art director from director Steven Spielberg's production company visited San Diego. A lab scene from the movie was based on the appearance of the San Diego Zoo's Frozen Zoo, and the Jurassic Park entrance gates were inspired by some of the gates on the grounds at the Wild Animal Park.

Dad recognized the potential risks of cloning. But when it came to applying the concept to saving endangered wildlife, he clearly felt that the benefits outweighed the risks. He was enthusiastic about learning and developing the techniques so they could be put to use. In 2000, when he was president of the Zoo's board of trustees, he arranged to send a vial of Frozen Zoo cells to Advanced Cell Technology (ACT), a biotechnology firm in Massachusetts. The cells were from a male gaur, a type of large wild ox. At the time, the number of gaur had dropped to less than 36,000 worldwide due to declines in its natural habitats in South and Southeast Asia. The gaur, listed as threatened, was on its way to becoming officially endangered. Dad wanted to see if cloning could help save this vulnerable species.

ACT inserted genetic material from the male gaur's cells into egg cells of common cows (where the original cow's genetic material had been removed). Forty embryos were then transferred into domestic cows, and eight viable pregnancies were detected. One gaur, named Noah, was carried to full term and born on January 8, 2001. Unfortunately, it died two days later from a common bacterial infection that was unrelated to cloning. Nevertheless, Dad and many other scientists were encouraged: the first attempt at cloning a threatened species had succeeded.

The next year, the San Diego Zoo provided cells to ACT from a male banteng, a wild ox native to Southeast Asia. Only about 8,000 bantengs remained in their native habitat at the time, making the species officially endangered. Once again, the genetic material was inserted into cow eggs, which were then implanted in 30 female cows. Sixteen pregnancies resulted, of which two went to term. Two calves were born in April 2003. One was twice the normal birth weight and had to be euthanized soon after birth. The remaining male banteng clone appeared healthy, although it was later determined that it had no functional testicular tissue so it couldn't pass on its genes. The cloned banteng became a symbol of hope for the successful cloning of endangered wildlife—as well as a reminder of the many challenges in staving off the extinction of species.

Despite the obstacles, Dad was still very optimistic that cloning could one day help to conserve wildlife. He wrote, "There is no doubt in my mind that the zoo world will have to learn how to clone their vanishing species. I'm hoping this will develop further from the specimens that we have collected—that is, to intentionally clone animals that are really in need of reproduction. I am convinced this will be practiced widely in the next 50 years." The fact that it was even possible to try was due to the efforts that my father and others had made in establishing the Frozen Zoo. Now, Dad's favorite quote from Daniel Boorstin seemed almost prophetic: "You must collect things for reasons you don't yet understand."

∞

The Frozen Zoo had grown to become an integral part of the San Diego Zoo's conservation research—so valuable that some staff members worried about it day and night. When Marlys Houck was hired in 1987, she joined Arlene Kumamoto in managing the collection of samples. At the time, the Frozen Zoo consisted of two liquid nitrogen freezers in the Scripps building, one freezer with original tissue samples and the other with duplicates. After hearing about the accidental 1977 thaw and the devastating loss of genetic material, Marlys had recurring nightmares about losing the collection to another thaw or fire. One night, she had an especially disturbing nightmare about the freezers breaking through the upstairs floor and landing on her bed.

"That does it!" Arlene said the next day when Marlys told her about the nightmare. "We have to move one of the freezers to another location." It took five years to get approval and a properly prepared site. Finally in 1992, the Frozen Zoo—by then expanded to four freezers, two with duplicate samples—was divided between the Scripps building and a warehouse on the other side of the Zoo.

In 1999, Marlys left her mark in another way. Up to that point, the Frozen Zoo had only stored the tissue of mammals, but Marlys was working on a project for identifying the sex of birds by growing cells from feathers. Once she was done with the cells, they were discarded. Arlene was concerned that the staff didn't have time for the complicated process of cataloging and freezing avian cells, so she never encouraged them to try to bank the cells in the Frozen Zoo. But Marlys believed that not saving the cells was a mistake. The next time Dad was in the office asking about what everyone was working on, Marlys pulled him aside to show him the bird cells under a microscope. "Look at my bird cells," she said. "Aren't they pretty?"

Dad peered through the lens. "Those are beautiful," he said. "You're putting them in the Frozen Zoo, aren't you?"

"Well, no," Marlys said innocently. "Arlene doesn't want me to. She says we have enough to do."

"Mushi! Get in here!" Dad called, using his pet name for Arlene, a term of endearment that is loosely translated from Japanese as "bug." When Arlene arrived, he said, "Look at these cells—they're beautiful. You need to help Marlys put them in the Frozen Zoo. We have to start saving these bird cells." And that was the beginning of the expansion of species in the Frozen Zoo, which now includes reptiles, amphibians, fish, and even plant seeds.

In 2004, the Frozen Zoo recorded another milestone. Over Thanksgiving weekend that year, the world's last living po'ouli—a black-faced honeycreeper native to Hawaii—died of old age at a conservation center on the island of Maui. Marlys received a call that the bird's body would be delivered to San Diego later that day. Because it was the last bird of its kind, the team had already planned to preserve the po'ouli's cells for the Frozen Zoo. The bird's feathers weren't suitable for growing cells, so any attempt at growing a cell line would have to come directly from tissue. The pressure was on, but after several stressful weeks, Marlys succeeded, banking cells from the first extinct bird in the Frozen Zoo. Ollie Ryder said of the bittersweet triumph, "We will never hear the po'ouli honeycreeper's song again, but we can learn from its genetic code."

Research can be a slow, painstaking process, but working to save extinct wildlife sometimes requires quick action. Lonesome George, a century-old Galápagos tortoise from Pinta Island in the Galápagos Islands chain, was the last of the La Pinta subspecies of giant Galápagos tortoises. He died of natural causes in 2012. Staff members there recognized the significance of the event and refrigerated his body so that George's tissue could be preserved. They contacted scientists from the Frozen Zoo in San Diego for advice on how to collect tissue appropriately, but they didn't have the proper reagents for the sample collection process. "Suddenly we realized that if one of us didn't go down there quickly to help, we would lose our last chance to save cells from this extraordinary animal," Marlys recalls. "So we scrambled, and within 24 hours, two of us were on a plane headed south for the Galápagos Islands."

The San Diego team arrived in time to process the samples, but because of permit issues, those samples had to remain behind. "One day we hope to bring them here, but the main point is that tissues were saved and are now preserved," Marlys says. "If we hadn't made the decision to go right then, that would have meant that the last, living parts of Lonesome George and his kind would've been gone—forever."

The Frozen Zoo played a key role in another advance that was reported in the scientific journal *Nature Methods* in 2011. Five years earlier, Japanese scientists had demonstrated that it was possible to convert nonreproductive cells into pluripotent stem cells—that is, master cells that could potentially develop into any type of cell or tissue. Some of those same scientists then showed it was possible to turn those induced cells into eggs and sperm. That meant a fertilized egg derived from ordinary skin cells might one day be placed in a surrogate mother, giving new life to an endangered species.

Building from this research, the 2011 paper, coauthored by Marlys, Ollie, and nine others, described the first time that induced pluripotent stem cells had been generated from endangered animals. The subjects were a mandrill (a primate related to baboons) and a northern white rhinoceros. The cells in both cases came from the Frozen Zoo. These breakthroughs showed that the prospect of rescuing wildlife with the help of banked tissue culture cells was becoming more and more real. My father's instinct to preserve tissue samples decades before was prescient. The new cases gave conservationists worldwide great hope that all was not lost.

In December 2019, a playful, three-week-old southern white rhinoceros at the San Diego Zoo Safari Park was happily taking advantage of a recent rainstorm to get down and dirty. As wildlife care specialist Marco Zeno explained at the time, the baby rhino's "new favorite thing is mud. She sees a puddle, and she just needs to roll in it!" The calf, aptly named Future, weighed nearly 200 pounds and was expected to reach up to 4,000 pounds when fully grown. But Future wasn't just any rhino baby—she was, and is, an important example of the latest conservation efforts involving the Zoo, its researchers, and its partner organizations.

The northern white rhinoceros, a close relative of the southern white rhino, is on the verge of extinction. The last male northern white rhino died in 2018, leaving just two females at a conservancy in Kenya. They are the final surviving members of their species in the entire world.

Hope for saving the northern white rhino, however, may still be alive. This hope may lie in cell cultures in the Frozen Zoo and with a dedicated international team of scientists and conservationists that includes the Zoo's Barbara Durrant. In 2019, scientists in Italy took eggs from the surviving two northern white rhino females and inseminated them in a lab with previously collected and frozen northern white rhino sperm—including samples saved in the Frozen Zoo. The resulting embryos were then frozen so that they might one day be implanted in surrogate southern white rhino mothers.

Before using the embryos, the process of artificial insemination needed to be tested. At the San Diego Zoo Safari Park, Barbara Durrant and her team worked with two female southern white rhinos at the Park's Nikita Kahn Rhino Rescue Center. One was artificially inseminated with frozen semen, a first in North America for this species. The other was inseminated with chilled semen—a first in the world for any rhino species. The team was thrilled when each mother successfully gave birth to a calf in 2019: Edward, as a result of the frozen semen, and Future, as a result of the chilled semen. The birth of these southern white rhino calves showed that the process could succeed.

It was a huge milestone, and it buoyed the team's hopes that they eventually might be able to apply similar techniques to helping save the northern white rhino. Refining the necessary steps in the artificial reproduction process is complex—it may be another 10 or 20 years before it's possible to attempt a northern white rhino birth with a surrogate mother—but the Zoo's scientists are cautiously optimistic that they will get there.

Long before almost anyone else, Dad recognized the significance of the Frozen Zoo and the potential of genetic advances such as cloning—and what they could mean for endangered wildlife and for human health. In his notes for a book, he wrote, "The recent production of cloned pigs in August 2000 raises the hope that one might raise genetically modified pigs [they have the closest biologic similarity to us] that could be donors of livers for patients needing transplants. Understanding how difficult it is to get organs for patients suffering from liver cancer, hepatitis C, and other diseases that affect the liver, you can easily understand how attractive such a prospect is. For the zoo world, this presents the possibility that one could produce animals that have become so scarce they might otherwise die out. Take an okapi; few exist. Or the Przewalski's horse, which has become extinct in the wild and now lives only in zoos around the world."

Twenty years later, Dad's predictions are again coming true. Today's scientists have already performed pig-to-human organ transplants. In recent years, advances in gene-editing technology have reduced the risks of organ rejection and transmitting porcine viruses. Some scientists are predicting that these transplants will be possible within the next few years, dramatically increasing the scarce supply of organs and potentially saving human lives around the world.

∞

Then there is the case of the Przewalski's horse. Dad had a special interest in this animal since the early 1960s, when he was the first person to determine that it had a different number of chromosomes than domestic horses. The Przewalski's horse was, he realized, a separate species and the last truly wild horse. In the 1970s, he passed that interest to Ollie Ryder, who made the Przewalski's horse a major focus of his research for decades.

During his years of study, Ollie made seven trips to the Askaniya–Nova Biosphere Reserve in Ukraine, which boasts the world's largest group of Przewalski's horses. While there, he worked with scientists and the animal care staff on how to manage and improve genetic diversity when such a limited number of animals existed. As a result of this work and a cooperative breeding program, the population of Przewalski's horses increased significantly, and the horses have now been reintroduced to their native habitat.

In 1980, Ollie received a skin biopsy from a five-year-old Przewalski's horse named Kuporovic, which he preserved in the Frozen Zoo. Forty years later, this stallion's genetic material was thawed and inserted into an egg from a female Przewalski's horse. Then, using the latest technology, the embryo was implanted into a surrogate mother, a domestic horse.

On August 6, 2020, a healthy Przewalski's foal was born to the surrogate mother at a veterinary facility in Texas. This was the first successful clone of a Przewalski's horse. Remarkable!

The team of scientists decided on a special name for this groundbreaking newborn: "Kurt." They wanted to honor Dad for everything he'd done to advance the understanding of genetics, the potential of cloning, and the importance of applying what we learn from human and veterinary medicine to saving wildlife like the Przewalski's horse. All of us in the Benirschke family were humbled when the Zoo called to tell us. We couldn't think of a more appropriate tribute to my father, whose namesake foal will live on and breed, helping to propagate future generations.

CHAPTER 23

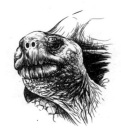

A Unique Individual

I t isn't easy to capture the essence of a man in a few words or even a few chapters—especially when that man is your father, and especially when he is as accomplished a man as Dr. Kurt Benirschke. Dad possessed a fascinating combination of qualities that allowed him to do remarkable things and made him a unique and influential person.

His incredible intellectual curiosity was one of his primary and most admirable traits, and it fueled his entire career. He never lost his enthusiasm for learning—about everything from science to music to how the world worked—and that insatiable curiosity and the ability to link ideas led him to make many new discoveries. Even when he was in his mid-80s, working in the morgue at UCSD, Dad said more than once to his friend Ken Jones, "Ken, I can't believe that there are still so many exciting questions to ask." Dad loved to talk to friends and colleagues about the latest breakthroughs in pathology, genetics, wildlife conservation, comparative medicine—or whatever else was on his mind.

He enjoyed sharing his passion for learning with everyone, regardless of title, background, beliefs, or bank account. As a young boy, I often accompanied Dad when he went into his lab at Dartmouth's medical school early on Saturday mornings. One day when I joined him, the halls were deserted except for the janitor, a man named Wayne, who was sweeping the floor.

"Wayne, how are you doing today?" Dad asked cheerfully and sincerely.

"Good morning, Dr. B," Wayne replied with equal warmth. "You're here early this morning."

Dad was so excited to be back in his lab that he almost couldn't help himself. "Wayne," he said, "do you want to see what I'm working on?" He beckoned the janitor over to a microscope, mounted a slide, and started describing his latest project as Wayne peered through the lens. I watched him repeat that scene countless times over the years with so many others. It didn't matter to my dad who you were or where you came from. He treated you like a person, with value.

Dad was known for asking good questions and for conducting research that expanded multiple fields of science. Like any good teacher, he enjoyed inspiring others to make their own discoveries. As Mary (Byrd) Cole explains, "He was always encouraging me to use my brain and taught me how to figure things out on my own. He showed me how to look at things in a different way." One of his favorite things to do at the Zoo was to encourage staff members to learn the taxonomic list of animal orders—and he was known to quiz them by asking them to recite it.

My father's hard-charging personality didn't endear him to everyone, particularly if you didn't show interest in what he was doing or talking about. But he was extremely generous with people in need and with anyone who truly wanted to learn. A high school student in Mississippi once wrote a letter asking if Dad could send her camel's blood for a research project. He wrote her back, explaining that camels were quite resistant to having their blood drawn and that he was sorry he wouldn't be able to help. A month later, however, a camel happened to die at the Zoo, so Dad asked Mary, "Would you find that letter from the high school girl?" He went on to contact the young student, explaining that because of an unforeseen situation, he could now send the blood sample if she could still use it.

"For a man in his position to remember a high school student in Mississippi and take that time is just one of many examples that showed how much he really cared about people," Mary says.

Dad was also generous with his students. In 1979, his student Bruce Rideout, an undergraduate at UCSD who was interested in veterinary medicine, was working in the Zoo's endocrine laboratory on a project involving reproductive issues in nine-banded armadillos. For the armadillo project, he sometimes needed Dad's help to interpret what he was seeing under the microscope.

One day, Bruce was waiting outside of Dad's office while a pathologist from UCSD's medical school discussed some of his latest slides with Dad. My father was hard on his colleague, saying, "Why are you misinterpreting this? This isn't what you think it is." As Bruce listened to the conversation, he wondered if he, a lowly undergrad, was in store for similar treatment—or worse.

But when his turn came, "Dr. B sat down with me and was as nice as he could possibly be," says Bruce. "He helped me understand what I was seeing in my slides. He was an internationally recognized expert and could have easily passed me on to someone else, but he took the time to work with me. It was great and made a big impact on me."

In fact, Dad helped launch Bruce's career by coauthoring one of his first scientific papers, "Stress-induced Adrenal Changes and Their Relation to Reproductive Failure in Captive Nine-banded Armadillos," published in 1985. For many years, Bruce occupied the same office in the Scripps building at the Zoo, serving as the director of disease investigations. He also became a diplomate of the American College of Veterinary Pathologists, an adjunct professor at San Diego State University, and a research fellow of the Peregrine Fund.

"Dr. B was super helpful to me," Bruce remembers. "If you were a student, he had unlimited time and energy for you. He once loaned a student his VW Bug for the summer. If he considered you a friend or respected colleague, or if you were a student, he would do anything to help you."

My father had high expectations of people, but he could also be gracious. In 1998, he was honored for his contributions to neonatology with the Virginia Apgar Award, named after the inventor of the Apgar score for assessing newborns in an attempt to combat infant mortality. Dad had actually met with Virginia Apgar several times to discuss their mutual interest in comparative biology. Frank Mannino, a UCSD neonatologist and good friend, had nominated Dad for the award and gave a speech and slide presentation at the ceremony. Following the event in San Francisco, Dad relayed his appreciation to Frank in a note: "There are no words to express my gratitude to you . . . but I am deeply touched by all of this and value your friendship enormously. Thanks."

At times, Dad's assistance went beyond work and careers. In December 1984, Doug Myers was the deputy director of the Zoological Society of San Diego and was soon to be named executive director. Six months before, Doug's wife had delivered their first child. The baby, a daughter named Amy, had been positioned upside down and backward in the womb and was born with a slight indentation in her skull. A couple of days earlier, doctors had recommended that Amy have surgery to correct the problem, but the issue wasn't obvious to Doug and his wife and they weren't sure what to do. To them, their daughter was already perfect.

On that day, Dad walked into Doug's office at the Zoo—he never knocked—and found Doug sitting at a table, staring into space. "What's wrong?" Dad asked.

Doug looked up. "Nothing's wrong. Everything's fine."

Dad shook his head. "No, I can tell by looking at you that something's wrong. What is it?"

Doug sighed and explained the situation with his daughter.

"Do you have a picture of her?" Dad asked. Doug did. My father looked at the photograph for a moment, turned it upside down, and showed it to Doug.

That simple visual shift changed everything. Suddenly, Doug could see what the doctors were talking about. "Okay," he said. "We need to get this thing taken care of."

Dad picked up the phone in Doug's office and started making calls. A few minutes later, he told Doug, "I just spoke to a Dr. Robinson in Philadelphia. He's the best in the world at this kind of surgery. You should call him right now." Doug did, and Dr. Robinson arranged for a colleague in San Diego—a former student—to perform the surgery on Amy's skull. Despite doctors' initial concerns about Amy's health and intellectual capacity, the surgery was a success, and she grew up to be an outstanding student and successful CPA, wife, and mother. Today, Doug gives Dad much of the credit for "helping to make my daughter healthy."

"When you have somebody that smart, that well connected, that passionate, that empathetic and caring on your side," Doug says, "you can't lose."

Something similar happened in 2002 when Amy Parrott, then director of individual and planned gifts at the Zoo, noticed that her 15-year-old daughter had unusual swelling on her right ankle. Initially, Laura and her mother weren't too concerned, but over the next six months, the swelling got worse and spread up Laura's leg to her knee. Doctors couldn't seem to diagnose the problem. When Amy asked Laura's doctor, "Isn't there anything else you can do?" his response was, "No."

"So, what do you do when no one else can figure out what's wrong?" Amy says with a grin. "You go talk to Dr. B."

Dad suggested that Amy send him a list of everything they'd learned and done about the situation, and he invited Amy and her daughter to come to the house that weekend. My brother, Steve, a respected orthopedist in Seattle, was coming for a visit and would be there too. They would "take a look," Dad said, and see what they could do.

The next Saturday afternoon, Amy, Laura, Steve, and Dad were gathered in the living room of my parents' house when Mom arrived with a guest. Marvin Jones, the Zoo's longtime registrar, was also having health issues and was being discharged from the hospital with no one to take care of him. Dad had offered to have Marvin stay with them. "The rest of us were all sitting there," Amy recalls, "while Dr. B was assisting Marvin up the stairs. It was chaos, but it was because of Dr. B's desire to help people."

Once Marvin was situated, Dad came down to talk with Steve about Laura's problem. They reached out to Ken Jones at UCSD to get his opinion, and then they sent an email to Dad's extensive medical contact list to see if anyone had experience with Laura's condition. They also copied information that Dad found in one of his books and gave it to Amy to read.

Dad concluded that Laura likely had lymphedema, a buildup of too much lymphatic fluid. It was an incurable but treatable condition. But to be certain, he told Amy she should see the "one doctor in the country who really knows this stuff." He helped them get in touch with the doctor, which resulted in a trip to Phoenix and a correct diagnosis of primary lymphedema. Laura eventually had successful surgery to remove the lymphatic fluid. As an adult, Laura wears custom-made support stockings to treat her condition and lives a normal life.

"I'm so eternally grateful that Dr. B took the time for us," Amy says. "It was a miracle to me that he was able to figure this out when no one else could. I'm afraid to think about what would have happened if I hadn't gone to see him."

Doug Myers adds: "Today, when I hear about people with medical problems, the first person that comes to mind is Dr. Benirschke. I think, 'If only I could call him. I'm sure he would know the answer.' He never gave up. He would either find the solution to your problem himself or find the person who knew the answer. He was an extraordinary guy."

My father had his idiosyncrasies. For one thing, whether he was helping someone or pursuing another scientific theory, he was always in a hurry. People had trouble keeping up with him when he was on foot and when he drove. He left a lot of people gasping for air when he took the hospital steps two at a time (he rarely rode an elevator), and he racked up a few speeding tickets behind the wheel as he motored from the hospital to the Zoo and back again.

One day in 2005, Dad was rushing to pick up something from the Scripps building at the Zoo, but he drove a little too fast into the parking lot and ended up denting another car's rear fender. When he dashed into the autopsy room, a lab technician who'd seen his parking mishap said, "Dr. B, I think you hit my car."

"Oh, that was your car?" Dad said apologetically. He wanted to pay for the damage, of course, but he was also in a hurry. He emptied his wallet and pockets of all the cash he had on him and thrust it into the technician's hands. "Here," he said, "this should take care of it. If not, you know where to find me." That was Dad.

My dad was stubborn, and that extended to his culinary choices. He was a picky eater who did not like vegetables and preferred the German specialties his mother had made when he was growing up. He was always thin, probably because he often missed lunch. Dad was always too busy and too absorbed in whatever he was doing to eat. He did love desserts, though, and usually had a foot-long bar of dark chocolate on his desk at the Zoo and medical center. He regularly carved off a chunk with his pocketknife and encouraged visitors to do the same.

Dad enjoyed museums, flowers, and novels by authors such as Kurt Vonnegut and Gabriel García Márquez, but he mostly spent his time reading medical journals. As in his youth, he continued to love opera, and despite being a man who rarely showed his emotions, he could tear up at the sound of his favorite music. Dad once said that if he hadn't been a scientist, he would have liked to become an orchestra conductor or a race car driver. None of us doubted that if he had, he would have been one of the best.

Another thing he liked to do was tease, and he loved it when people could keep up with him. Behind the playful banter, however, was genuine admiration and respect that helped him forge strong friendships with his coworkers.

Never much for rules, he sometimes flouted requirements. Bruce Rideout recalled that in the autopsy room, Dad never wanted to bother with wearing safety gloves or the other protective attire that had become standard. He was from a generation of doctors who were careful but didn't worry much about contracting diseases. As Dad once tried to explain, he needed to feel the texture of placenta tissue to measure its health and "you lose that feel when you wear gloves." Bruce often walked into the autopsy room to find him at work on an animal, a pipe in his mouth, his tie thrown over his shoulder, wiping bloody hands on his apron. If Bruce chastised him, Dad waved it off. "I don't have time for that," he'd say, feigning annoyance. "I've got to be back at UCSD in a minute."

It was a different story, however, with pathology technician April Gorow. When an animal was born at the Zoo, April called Dad so he could come over and examine the placenta. She found him in the autopsy room without gloves, a mask, or scrubs. "Dr. B, you have to wear gloves! If you don't, you're going to get *me* in trouble!" she said.

He shot April a mock-indignant look and said, "You don't know what you're talking about."

"I know," April said. "But you don't want to get me in trouble, do you? If another doctor were to come in here and see you doing this, it wouldn't be good for me."

Dad sighed and slowly put on the gloves, making a show of it to communicate his disapproval. After he finished his work, he even stepped into the footbath to sterilize the bottom of his shoes—stomping his feet when he stepped out to make sure April noticed. This was an often-repeated scene in the years to come. The theatrical, reluctant cooperation was his way of showing respect, even affection.

Arlene Kumamoto was another coworker Dad highly respected and appreciated. As a UCSD graduate and one of the original members of the research team, Arlene engaged in many studies and authored dozens of papers with him on the genetic makeup of different endangered wildlife. She became an international authority on mammalian chromosomes, in addition to her duties managing the Frozen Zoo, and she was someone Dad leaned on often.

Dad and Arlene grew close during their nearly 25 years of working together. For my father's retirement from UCSD, Arlene expressed her appreciation by writing, "With love and gratitude for your guidance and friendship." It touched him deeply. Dad once said that the three women who had most shaped his life were Mom, Mary, and Arlene. It was a shock for him and everyone else who knew Arlene when, in September 1999, she began having abdominal pain and was diagnosed with an aggressive cancer. Arlene's health declined very quickly. Dad often visited her in the hospital, and when he saw her for the last time on January 7, 2000, he said she looked like a ghost. She died three days later at age 46. She left a hole at the research center, at the Zoo, and in the hearts of her loved ones and colleagues—especially in Dad's—that could never be filled.

In 2007, Dad had the chance to fulfill one of his lifelong ambitions. He'd always wanted to visit the Galápagos Islands, where Charles Darwin collected samples in 1835 and made observations that led to his groundbreaking book, *On the Origin of Species*. Knowing that Dad was approaching his mid-80s, Mary (Byrd) Cole organized a 10-day trip for him that included a chartered boat. The 16-member party included Dad; Mary and her family; Ingrid and her husband, Gordon; and Dad's former colleague Mark Bogart. I was unable to take time off work and could not go, a regret I still carry. Dad enjoyed the trip immensely, seeing the natural wildlife that included the enormous Galápagos tortoises and visiting the Charles Darwin Research Station on Santa Cruz Island.

Unfortunately, on that trip, he didn't want to bother with protection from the intense sun. With some arm-twisting, Ingrid and others eventually managed to persuade him to wear a hat and sunglasses, but Dad refused to put on sunscreen. As Mary says, "He thought he could defy the sun." The result was "the worst sunburn you've ever seen," especially on his knees and legs. Dad could barely walk, but he never complained and wouldn't admit that he was in pain. Nonetheless, it was a trip he loved and talked about often.

Even in his late 80s, Dad continued to stop in at UCSD to examine interesting placentas and take calls from scientists at the Zoo's conservation research center whenever his knowledge or wisdom was needed. That changed in March 2012 when he suffered a second heart attack and a stroke.

The stroke was a big blow. He didn't have any paralysis, but the damage to his brain left him with expressive aphasia, essentially taking away his ability to write, read, and speak. Even after weeks of speech therapy, he struggled with putting words together. Our family had to move Dad and Mom, who was also starting to have health issues, to an assisted living facility in La Jolla. We thought it would be a devastating turn for a man who was accustomed to making speeches to large audiences and writing complex scientific papers. But in the months and years that followed, Dad seemed to accept his new condition. He went on walks along the coast and enjoyed the various outings the assisted living facility put together for its residents. He developed enough verbal ability to offer a friendly "Hi, how are you?" greeting to other residents and to enjoy dinners with his new friends.

To Ingrid, our father became a changed man. She had always desired a closer relationship with him, and now she got her wish. She became the one who spent the most time helping Mom and Dad, assisting with everything from managing their medicines and paying their bills to hiring the nursing support they needed. "He became much softer and sweeter. He was more appreciative," Ingrid says, tearing up. "All he could do were visual things, so when I came to visit, we'd watch TV or movies together, and he would hold my hand. He was warm toward me, which took my breath away. Our relationship changed completely. I got so much closer to him in those last years. I felt it was a gift."

Dad had other visitors too, friends and colleagues like Ollie Ryder, Frank Mannino, Nancy Czekala, Marlys Houck, Tom Fetter, and many others. Ingrid tried to limit the visitors and the time they were there, because it was hard for Dad to speak and it could become uncomfortable for him and his guests. It was different, however, with Dave Fagan. The veterinary dentist had become one of Dad's most faithful friends and had seen him almost without fail at least once a week for four decades. Dave continued to visit my dad every Saturday, even after Dad moved into assisted living. Sometimes he took Dad for a drive along the coast, out for a beer, to the Zoo, or on some other outing they decided upon on the spur of the moment. Other times Dave just sat with Mom and Dad on the patio outside their room, looking at the ocean and the passersby. Dave did most of the talking, of course, but Dad genuinely appreciated the company. All of us kids will never be able to thank Dave enough for how much his visits meant to us.

Dad's final overseas trip was in 2012, several months after the stroke, when he, Steve, and Mary traveled one last time to Paraguay to check on the status of his peccaries. As always, the trip included time in Filadelfia, one of his favorite places on Earth.

After five years of living with frustrating physical limits, my father—who had always been so optimistic—found his spirits dimming. It became harder and harder for him to walk, and his body began giving out; we all knew his time was short. On September 10, 2018, Kurt Benirschke took his last breath and died peacefully. The official cause of death was congestive heart failure, but really, he was just ready to go. He was 94 years old.

The week before his death, I felt the impulse to bring him and Mom back to the Zoo for one more visit. Ingrid and I alerted the Zoo's leadership of our plans, and they surprised us by gathering a few of his closest colleagues and favorite animals and put together an informal "welcome back" event. After a brief ceremony, we put Dad in a wheelchair and pushed him around the Zoo to visit some of his favorite places.

As the news spread that he was on-site, staff members from across the Zoo found out where he was and came to greet him. There were lots of hugs and smiles and plenty of tears. Many staff members told Ingrid and me tender stories about something special that Dad had done for someone or some fun memory they had made together. It was touching for us, and everyone's kindness really moved Dad; he seemed to understand the impact he had on the Zoo and so many of the people there. It was a day we felt privileged to be able to share with him and Mom, and the photos are now so precious to us.

With Dad's death, we lost a much-loved and respected husband, father, and leader—a man who taught us the value of life in its many forms and how to live that life with integrity, curiosity, passion, and respect for others. The scientific and zoological worlds lost a visionary researcher, teacher, mentor, and champion of conservation. He is missed every day, but his impact lives on.

Mom was overcome with sorrow at the loss of her beloved companion of 66 years, often saying, "I'm ready to go and want to join him." She passed away peacefully just seven months later, on April 16, 2019. Both had chosen to be cremated, and Ingrid had promised Mom that when the time came, we would combine their ashes so they could be together forever.

A short time after their passing, our family and about 40 friends gathered on a catamaran in the San Diego Harbor, headed a mile off the coast in the Pacific Ocean, and launched Dad and Mom on their final voyage in a biodegradable cremation urn made in the shape of a whale. For almost five minutes, the papier-mâché whale bobbed gently on the surface. The sun glinted off the brilliant blue sea, and we scattered rose petals in the water. Ingrid later told me that she thought, "This is just right for Dad to be in the belly of a whale together with Mom at the end of their journey. He's surely smiling right now."

A minute later, the whale appeared to rise up, as if preparing to dive. Then it slowly disappeared beneath the surface, on course to mingle with the denizens of the deep.

EPILOGUE

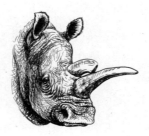

Legacy

After my father's death, Ollie Ryder wrote about him in the *Journal of Heredity*: "His impacts in the fields of genetics, pathology, medicine, and conservation are testaments to his special mix of scientific acumen, curiosity, focused commitment, and charismatic charm." Over the course of his long career, Dad authored or coauthored 30 books, close to 100 chapters in other books, and more than 500 scientific papers. His research and pioneering efforts had far-reaching effects on multiple fields of science during his lifetime. But his influence did not stop there.

Dad did not adhere to a formal religion, accepting but not sharing Mom's Catholic faith or the belief that I developed as a result of my struggles with illness. He believed, "You live your life, do the best you can to make a difference, and then it's just over and you're gone." His friend Dr. Frank Mannino has another view, though.

"I feel he was wrong about that," Frank says. "Kurt lives on in so many people around the world—pathologists, neonatologists, conservationists, and more. His legacy is ongoing."

One example of Dad's continuing influence is his website on comparative placentation. The website will be updated and expand on what he started, providing a significant resource for future veterinary pathologists and zoo veterinarians.

Then there is the Zoo's ongoing conservation research. The research center that Dad founded in the 1970s has helped grow the Zoo into an international leader for saving wildlife. The Arnold and Mabel Beckman Center for Conservation Research is home to eight research teams focused on population sustainability, recovery ecology, community engagement, disease investigations, conservation genetics, reproductive sciences, plant conservation, and biodiversity banking, and employs a total staff of 260.

The impact of the Frozen Zoo, part of the Zoo's Wildlife Biodiversity Bank, has grown to a level that only Dad could have imagined. It hosts viable cell cultures and gametes from more than 10,000 animals representing nearly 1,200 rare and endangered species and subspecies. Each is labeled and recorded with a "KB" (which stands for "Kurt Benirschke") lab number. Scientific investigators around the globe have benefited from approximately 7,000 samples the bank has provided, and the bank continues to offer a rich and ever-expanding resource for research and conservation. Conservation research staff members are also working with partners to support cryobanking efforts worldwide. At the Wildlife Biodiversity Bank today, there is a copy of the plaque that Dad originally posted near the collection, which includes his favorite quote about collecting from Daniel Boorstin. Nearby is another plaque bearing Dad's picture and a quote from him: "I don't think we have the right to say the world is made for us alone."

My father's efforts to bridge the gap between human and animal medicine also continue to bear fruit. The One Medicine movement, now referred to as One Health, is gaining momentum around the world and has been formally endorsed by the United States, the European Commission, the United Nations, the World Health Organization, and many others. In San Diego, UCSD medical faculty continue to volunteer their expertise at the Zoo and Safari Park, developing new healthcare techniques that benefit both animals and humans. In 2020, for example, an ophthalmologist for humans performed cataract surgery on a gorilla.

Dad was a master at assembling the leading authorities on a given topic so that people could meet face to face at a conference and discuss new ideas and ways to collaborate. Ollie Ryder has continued the tradition. In 2019, Ollie organized a meeting in San Diego of international experts in conservation genetics, reproductive physiology, sociology, ethics, law, cryobiology, and conservation biology. They discussed the progress, obstacles, and ramifications of the northern white rhino conservation project, including ethical and social issues. It was a gathering that may serve as a model for future discussions of wildlife conservation, and it was an event that Dad would have loved.

My father "raised" a generation of researchers and scientists to think and share the way he did—to keep asking questions, to challenge conventional wisdom and authority, to anticipate the future and consider long-term implications, and to cooperate and publish so that discoveries can be known and that understanding can expand. Those researchers and scientists are now mentoring another generation. His influence is spreading in an ever-widening circle.

It seems that Dad inspired a desire to question and learn more in almost everyone he encountered. Bill Lasley, professor emeritus at the UC Davis School of Veterinary Medicine and Center for Health and the Environment as well as primate assay core lead at the California National Primate Research Center, believes that this was one of my father's greatest gifts.

"Kurt taught that it's not enough to recognize that something happens. That's not the end of the story," Bill says. "The end of the story is when you figure out *how* and *why* something happens. Most people don't burden themselves with mental exercises in the unknown. They have to learn that way of thinking, and

Kurt was uniquely capable of teaching it. I'm still chasing some of the conundrums that he presented to me."

∞

Though he was always eyeing new goals and discoveries, Dad found his career and life highly fulfilling. On reflection, he remained grateful that he had the opportunity to come to America. His new home country gave him the opportunity to explore both medical and veterinary disciplines. He was also pleased with his career choice of pathology and focus on the placenta. "The placenta is not an organ that many pathologists have taken very seriously," Dad once said. "If I were to classify tumors of the thyroid or of the breast, I'd become a better-known pathologist. But I don't mind. The placenta is much more interesting, at least to me."

In 1988, he gave the commencement address to the graduating class at Dartmouth's medical school. In his final remarks, he gave advice to the graduates—words of wisdom he had clearly followed himself: "If you really want to, you can do anything in this great country, anything that is given to you by your smarts and by your will. All you have to do is trust in yourself, continue with the learning process, and be of good cheer."

Dad was devoted to his family as well as his career. What he struggled to say to us in person he was able to verbalize in a TV interview: "I love my family. I'm deeply indebted to them for allowing me to pursue all my interests." He was grateful for his frequent opportunities to travel and see the world. But he said that, like Robert Browning wrote in his poem "Home-Thoughts, from Abroad," he too yearned for home when away.

Dad had lived, he once said, an "exciting life." When asked in an interview how he would like to be remembered, he had a simple answer: as the savior of the *taguá*, the peccary of Paraguay. That was Dad. He could have listed all manner of accomplishments, but he didn't like to talk about his achievements in a self-congratulatory way. He was a big thinker with a simple but important philosophy, one that was perhaps captured best by another favorite quote, attributed to Chief Seattle:

> What is man without the beasts? If all the beasts were gone, man would die from a great loneliness of the spirit. For whatever happens to the beasts, soon happens to man. All things are connected.

More than most people, Dad saw those connections—between humans and animals, between scientific theory and practical application, between making the most of the present and keeping an eye toward the future, between generously sharing time and insights and receiving the benefits of that sharing for all. Dad was the modern version of a Renaissance man. I doubt that we will see anyone quite like him again. We miss him.

AFTERWORD

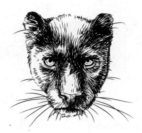

It Takes All of Us

In October 2019, I had the honor of taking over the leadership reins of San Diego Zoo Global and guiding an organization that has been truly transformed by Dr. Benirschke's vision and desire for impact. The groundwork he laid over his years here cannot be overstated: his efforts have helped set up our organization for its next chapter.

On March 3, 2021, World Wildlife Day, we announced the evolution of our organization into San Diego Zoo Wildlife Alliance—a change that was empowered by a core belief I formed during 2020 as the world endured a global pandemic. This rebranding was much more significant than a change in our name. I realized we could, and should, do more to protect wildlife around the world. We had more than a century of experience and incredible talent across our organization in conservation science, wildlife care, health, and nutrition. We needed to be more strategic in how we worked. And we needed to more fully communicate and represent our role as one of the world's leading zoos in global conservation.

To do this, we would have to listen to the needs of people and wildlife, just as Dr. B did when asking the team how he could help. This would be essential if we were to truly help drive greater outcomes for wildlife. We would also need to change how we showed up in the field—how we worked with partners and fellow conservation organizations.

Dr. B was a pioneer of the One Medicine concept. This groundbreaking approach has evolved today into the larger scientific community's One Health movement, which focuses on identifying the interconnectedness of wildlife, ecosystems, and people. This may have seemed like an obscure thought to the public prior to the events that unfolded in 2020, but I am confident that by now, we all have a much better appreciation for the need to keep in better balance with nature.

Dr. B was ahead of his time in thinking the organization should collect DNA and tissue samples and keep them in what is today our Wildlife Biodiversity Bank. We are thankful he did. It was his vision that currently enables San Diego Zoo Wildlife Alliance to make strides in bringing back the northern white rhino, and in 2020 allowed us to be an integral part of welcoming two clones from endangered species: Kurt, a Przewalski's horse, and Elizabeth Ann, a black-footed ferret. Because of Dr. B's foresight and his help, we have enough genetic diversity to truly change the trajectory for a species.

It was this kind of visionary approach that drew people to Dr. B and inspired them to join him here. They were drawn to his bold desire to change the world. It is in that same spirit that we at San Diego Zoo Wildlife Alliance must continue to evolve how we work. If we are going to carry that torch forward, we must continue to innovate just as he did. And we must help, because the challenges facing wildlife are too great for any one organization or approach to solve alone.

The wildlife conservation community started pursuing a One Medicine strategy long before it was publicly discussed, because wildlife conservationists had known for some time that everything was—and is—interconnected. We cannot protect wildlife unless the local community wants to protect the species with which they coexist. The community must see the value and importance of doing so. People need to see how protecting species makes their lives and the lives of their families better. Only then can we effectively bring other skills to the table to support wildlife conservation.

And this is where San Diego Zoo Wildlife Alliance stands uniquely tall. Few, if any, organizations have the experience and knowledge that we have gained from operating the world-famous San Diego Zoo since 1916 and the San Diego Zoo Safari Park since 1972. The depth of our skill set is unmatched in caring for wildlife, which makes us a powerful partner for other wildlife conservation organizations. Many of them are premier habitat and ecosystems experts, but they could benefit from our organization's extensive wildlife knowledge and expertise when pursuing a One Health strategy in the field.

I think back to Dr. Benirschke going around to each team at the Zoo and Park and asking, "What challenges can I help to solve or address?" At the time, his approach was groundbreakingly collaborative. We need to support all conservationists and encourage them to embrace a collaborative approach to their work. No single scientist will solve the issues facing wildlife alone. Collaboration always accelerates innovation. If we care about outcomes, we must care about how we can effectively drive change. Innovation only matters as much as it can be built upon, communicated, and scaled. Albert Einstein taught us that. A One Health approach requires collaboration as the first order. We all must be humble supporters, drivers, and instigators of change. I say *humble* because ego has no place in conservation. Impact and outcomes do. I can think of few people who understood this more than Dr. Benirschke from his simple and essential approach of, "How can I help?"

Our name change to San Diego Zoo Wildlife Alliance lays out how we will pursue our conservation work in the future. The word *Alliance* is there for a reason. It will take all of us working together both as individuals and groups—helping one another; collaborating with different conservation organizations, leading partners, and local communities; and bringing forward our unique skills to the field of wildlife conservation.

I have a famous quote sitting on my desk that can be seen by all who enter my office. It reads: "There is no limit to what one can achieve as long as they don't mind who gets the credit." Dr. Benirschke was committed to changing the world, and he did not care who got the credit as long as they changed the world.

There is no doubt in my mind that if Dr. Benirschke were with us today, he would continue to insist, if not demand, that we reach for our full potential as an organization. To do that today means training and teaching our own scientists, conservationists, care specialists, and the rest of our teams to ask, "How can we scale our expertise? How can we share our knowledge to empower our team members and partners in the field to protect and save wildlife more effectively? How can we teach and mentor the next generation so they have more tools earlier in their careers? How can we work together to find more comprehensive solutions by bringing our various skills to the table in service to the community and wildlife?"

How can *we* help?

At San Diego Zoo Wildlife Alliance, we often say that effective conservation starts with people. Few have understood that better than Dr. Benirschke. And it's his powerful legacy we get to build upon as we reach to meet our full potential in our next chapter.

Paul A. Baribault
President and Chief Executive Officer
San Diego Zoo Wildlife Alliance

ACKNOWLEDGMENTS

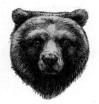

Dad's diverse interests led him to interact with colleagues and friends from around the world. He left his mark on their lives, and they in turn touched him. Many of these people generously shared their time and memories for this book; no doubt hundreds more would have if time and space allowed it. To each of them, I offer my heartfelt thanks.

Though it simply isn't possible to personally identify everyone who contributed in some way to this project, I do want to express particular appreciation to the following people: Allison Alberts, Chuck Bieler, Mark Bogart, Nancy Czekala, Barbara Durrant, Dave Fagan, April Gorow, Ken Jones, Bill Lasley, Frank Mannino, Dennis Meritt, Doug Myers, Amy Parrott, Dolores Pretorius, Bob Resnik, and Bruce Rideout. Special thanks also goes to Beth Autin and everyone on the staff at the San Diego Zoo Wildlife Alliance Library—including Ariel Hammond as well as Lisa Bissi from creative services—for diligently tracking down archival data and details. Marlys Houck deserves extra thanks for providing valuable insight and patiently answering repeated questions about the Frozen Zoo. And appreciation goes to Donna Armstrong, Albert Lund, and Laura McConnell for their comments on early chapter drafts.

I am especially grateful for the contributions and guidance of two of Dad's longtime colleagues and dear friends: Ollie Ryder and Mary (Byrd) Cole. I appreciate you both! I am also thankful to Paul Baribault, CEO of San Diego Zoo Wildlife Alliance, for his leadership in advancing the work my dad and his colleagues started by passionately focusing on conservation and endangered species.

Of course, Dad's family knew him best. This book would not have happened without the invaluable contributions of my sister, Ingrid, and my brother, Steve, along with my wife, Mary, and daughter, Kari. Thank you from the bottom of my heart for helping me honor Dad in this way.

Like any book, there are behind-the-scenes contributors who make it all happen, and for this book it was Georgeanne Irvine, Betsy Holt, Jim Lund, and my assistant, Patti McCord. Their love and respect for my dad and care for me were evident in the countless hours they spent making sure all the interviews were collected, the manuscript read and re-read so many times, photos gathered, and the myriad details checked and rechecked. Truly, this project would not have been completed without their dedication and commitment. Thank you.

Finally, to everyone who knew and loved my dad, thank you for being part of his remarkable story. If he were still with us today, he would thank you too.

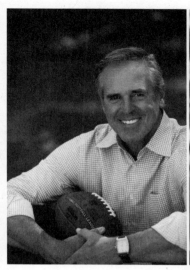
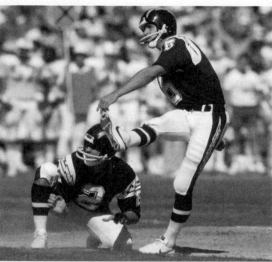

Rolf Benirschke

As a zoology major at UC Davis, Rolf Benirschke had a passion for wildlife and worked during his summers at the San Diego Zoo's Center for Reproduction of Endangered Species, the conservation division founded by his father, Dr. Kurt Benirschke. Following his graduation, Rolf became an NFL placekicker. His career was nearly derailed during his third season by a life-threatening battle with ulcerative colitis that required two emergency surgeries six days apart. After a miraculous comeback, Rolf returned to play seven more seasons with the San Diego Chargers, earning numerous honors, including Walter Payton NFL Man of the Year, NFL Comeback Player of the Year, and All-Pro. He played in the Pro Bowl and became the 20th player inducted into the Chargers Hall of Fame. During his time in the NFL, Rolf also launched Kicks for Critters, a fundraising and awareness program to support the Zoo's wildlife conservation efforts.

Following his NFL career, Rolf dedicated his life to supporting patients. He is CEO of Legacy Health Strategies, a patient engagement company, and founder of the Grateful Patient Project. As a respected leader and speaker in the health care industry, Rolf works tirelessly as a patient advocate and is active in supporting legislation that encourages research and innovation and protects patients. He is the author of four books, including his autobiography, *Alive & Kicking*. In addition, he sits on the board of trustees at San Diego Zoo Wildlife Alliance. Rolf is married to the love of his life, Mary. They have four children, including three with special needs.

JAMES LUND

James Lund is an award-winning collaborator, editor, and author who enjoys helping people develop their voice and message. He is a publishing veteran who has worked with bestselling authors, public figures, and ministry leaders, including Max Lucado, George Foreman, Kathy Ireland, Tim Brown, Bruce Matthews, and Jim Caviezel. A former newspaper journalist and book editor, Jim works on projects that range over a variety of themes and topics, from faith, adventure, risk, sports, and the military to marriage, parenting, business, and music. His work has taken him across the country and around the world, including to Kabul, Afghanistan. Book sales from Jim's projects exceed three million copies. Three have earned the Evangelical Christian Publishers Association Gold Medallion Award. Jim lives in Oregon, where he enjoys hiking, softball, and performing music with friends.